INSIDE OUT WEIGHT MANAGEMENT

Overcoming Emotional Eating and Breaking the Cycle of Yo-Yo Dieting

By Meg Cline

Table of Content

Chapter 1: My Story

Baltimore, October 2004

The year I lived in Baltimore I struggled with my weight more than I ever had before. This was especially maddening because after a year long journey to lose weight, I was finally where I wanted to be and was trying to maintain it. I *thought* that this would be the easy part. The fun part - where I reaped the reward of all that hard work. The year before I had set out to lose the 30 pounds I had picked up on my 5'5" frame over the course of the last 3 years. I had lost it the right way – exercising four or five times a week and counting every calorie of every morsel I ate. But despite being at, or at least "close enough," to my goal weight, I still thought about food and struggled with my choices all the time.

I was tired of it.

I read books, blogs, and magazine articles – anything I could find about weight loss. I ran longer, kept less food in the house and tried to distract myself when I felt those overwhelming food cravings rear up. The struggle to maintain my new weight was consistent, and followed me through graduation, a new boyfriend, moving twice and a new job. Many happy events in my life were clouded by the subconscious turmoil over my weight.

My story of weight gain and loss isn't particularly unusual or even that interesting when I compare it to many of the stories and long histories I've heard over the years from my clients. But there's a common thread that runs through every weight loss story and my story is no exception. The unhappiness I felt as I noticed the scale creep up seemed to permeate so many aspects of my life and began to fold itself into my identity. I have found that this overwhelming presence in the mind about "my weight" becomes true for almost everyone, whether they have 12 pounds or 152 pounds to lose and it helps explains the difficulty of making long term changes.

I can't exactly pinpoint when I started carrying more weight than I was comfortable with, but I can remember the point that I decided I wanted to do something about it. I had never been extremely athletic throughout childhood and much preferred to sit and read a book over playing a rousing game of neighborhood capture the flag, but a combination of cheerleading and dance, good family eating habits and probably some fortuitous teenage metabolism kept everything in check until college.

I started running shortly after I got to college – an experience that proved to be both humbling and satisfying – and eventually worked my way into a gym and added in regular strength training and other types of workouts. As a self-described "non athlete," I was surprised at how much I loved pushing my physical limits in the gym or on the road, and I eventually decided to major in Health & Exercise Science as well as become a certified personal trainer.

During the summer in between my sophomore and junior year, I landed an internship at Duke University's corporate wellness program. I spent that summer working side by side with an amazing mentor, Lauren, an exercise physiologist who had been a college track star and was a regular marathon runner. I helped her launch an inaugural run/walk program where we introduced non-runners to a 5k training program and over the course of the summer, took them from couch potatoes to 5k finishers. I fell in love with helping other people meet their fitness goals and overcome health obstacles and knew I was working in the right field. Personally, I spent that summer training for my first sprint triathlon with Lauren's support and later that fall, while studying abroad in Spain, ran a marathon with my roommate Rachel through the beautiful wine country region of Bordeaux.

All of that doesn't exactly sound like the history of someone who would find themselves struggling with her weight, which is exactly why it was such a shock when I stepped on the scale after returning from my adventures in Spain and realized I had put on exactly 30 pounds from the day I stepped on to campus two and half years ago. To this day, the image of those numbers on the scale and the reeling sense I felt as they cruelly blinked back up at me is burned in my memory.

I had realized my weight was creeping up long before I stepped on the scale that winter day. Despite my regular exercise routine, I knew that many of the "excesses" that went along with a college lifestyle, such as the bag of candy corn I'd take with me to the library to study, or the bagel I'd grab for breakfast, the meals out with friends at cheap Mexican places where we'd eat ourselves silly on the free chips and salsa or of course, the weekend beers, were not doing any favors to my waistline. Of course, I tried to balance out these guilty pleasures with healthier choices when I could – I regularly visited our campus salad bar, measured out my favorite snack into one ounce servings in Ziploc bags (the original "100 calorie packs") and avoided fast food. But obviously my "balanced" approach to eating and my regular exercise routine weren't enough to counteract my weight slowly creeping up. The evidence was there. Even when I avoided the scale, my clothes wouldn't allow me to deny what was happening.

The first time I talked about this with someone was with the exercise physiologist I was working with at Duke, Lauren. We were out on a training run together and I mentioned how it bothered me that I felt like I kept gaining weight even though I worked out all the time and ate healthy. I actually expected her to say what any other girlfriend would have likely said when another woman brings up weight. But instead of the general platitudes of, "don't worry, you look fine!" or, "I'm sure it's not as much as you think it is!" she looked right at me and said, "If you think you're gaining weight, why don't you try writing down your food and see how much you're eating? It's probably more than you think."

I was admittedly a bit stunned at first. I hadn't expected her to agree with me, much less to accuse me of eating more than I claimed. Lauren, however, was one of the most kind and loving friends I had and I knew her words came from a place of trying to help, so I put my pride aside and started asking questions. And it turned out to be exactly what I needed to hear.

The first time I wrote down my foods and tracked the calorie count, I was shocked to see I took in an average of 3,000 calories. I didn't eat fast food or drink regular soda. I packed my lunches and cooked most of my meals at home. It was amazing to me how quickly the calories from snacking on Wheat Thins while watching *Friends* reruns or margaritas out with my friends added up.

Now that I understood the simple process of calories in and calories out, I expected to easily get a handle on my eating and get back to a healthier weight. It seemed like a pretty straightforward math problem and I knew had the tools to solve the equation: a pen, a notebook, a book with calorie counts and a hefty dose of motivation. It worked.

For about a week.

I didn't find tracking my calories to be particularly difficult, but I found sticking to my self-imposed goal of 1300 to be challenging some days and downright impossible on other days. Tracking gave me a sense of control, although I often felt despondent that I *lacked* the control to make healthier choices or missed my mark time and time again.

It took returning from Spain and seeing that 30 pound mark on the scale to make me get really serious about tracking my calories and trying to lose weight. When I returned to school in January, I became diligent about writing down what I ate – and more importantly, *changing* what I ate. Finally, things began to click and the scale began to reflect my efforts. I didn't return to my pre-college weight, but by the time summer rolled around I had lost about 20 pounds and was back to a healthy weight for my body.

It'd be nice if this was where my weight loss story ended, but unfortunately it was not. While I had seemingly mastered the key to managing my weight – eating a certain number of calories and exercising a certain number of minutes – I still felt the very real *presence* of that struggle, day in and day out. A year later, as I graduated college and moved into an apartment in Baltimore, I felt like I was fighting more than ever to maintain my weight.

It wasn't three years later, in October of 2007 that I began to feel comfortable with my weight, and confident that I would maintain it. Leading up to this point, I had completed my master's degree, moved from Baltimore to North Carolina and started a dream job coaching people on weight loss in a huge clinical research trial. Once I was entrenched day in and day out in the inner workings of weight loss, it seemed even more imperative that I set a good example on how to lose weight and how to keep it off. I figured the weight I had been staying at, with some minor ups and downs, was my "set point." I also assumed I would absolutely have to keep a food log for the rest of my life and that it was just normal to fight the constant up and down battle of stress-eating a box of Wheat Thins from time to time with a four mile run.

I can tell you exactly when the shift finally happened. When I stopped constantly fighting myself. When all of this suddenly became a whole lot...dare I say... easier. But more importantly, I'll tell you *how* it happened. And even better? How you can make it happen, too.

Rochester, December 2007

6

We were flying home from Christmas vacation spent with my family in Rochester, NY. When I reflect back on this moment, I can remember looking out the window and for a half second feeling like we were suspended, rather than moving through the air. That half-second occurred right as I held my pen, hesitantly, over the pages of my journal wondering whether I should commit in ink what I was about to say. I wrote:

> "I want to declare something. I am
> hesitant to even write it. But... it would
> seem that I have finally won a battle. A
> battle I have been waging for probably 9
> years. It is tempting to say, with my
> typical caution that it is just in remission
> and it could resurface at any point. But I
> am coming to believe in the power of
> thoughts and that our reality is built by
> the words we choose to write our
> thoughts. So, I will write it here, in
> pen. The battle is over. It will not come
> into 2008 with me. I am at peace with my
> body. I am healthy. I am a healthy eater. I
> am in control but not controlling. I am
> okay, right where I am. I am a good role
> model. I am *healthy*. It feels so good to
> declare that. It is a relief. I have been
> fighting this battle too long. I am weary
> and frustrated. But that battle was
> against *me*. I was trying to defeat me."

The tide had started turning in late fall. I had begun to practice being kinder to myself. I spoke to myself as I would to my clients, with encouraging words and patience. I told myself I was already what I wanted to be. "I am what I want to be. I am healthy. I am a healthy eater. I am in control but not controlling. I am a good role model." This was my new mantra.

It is a relief to me still to this day to read those words. In them, I can hear the mixture of joy, caution and relief I felt as I realized I had arrived at a moment that I had previously thought I'd never experience.

This entry was a far cry from a previous one, written 18 months before (August 2006):

> "Blah blah blah blah. That sums up how I feel. Why am I feeling so crappy? I should be happy – I'm healthy, I have a job, I've got health insurance, I'm not living long distance from my boyfriend. I'm unhappy with my self right now – mainly my body and the way I'm taking care of it. Which is so stupid because I've been working out all the time and eating good like 80% of the time. I've gained at least 5 pounds since I moved from DC [3 months] but I feel like I keep putting on clothes and they're tight. ... I know why I'm not losing weight, I keep doing my calories and I'm over like every day. How the hell am I supposed to get 300 people to stick to diets if I can't stick to mine? Every day I wake up and think today I will do it, today I will come in under my calories. I make plans, I spend way too much money on produce, I work my butt off at the gym and then I blow it, every day. I get upset, I eat recklessly. We have friends over or

go out, I want to enjoy myself. I get sick of veggies, I eat too many snacks and by 4 pm, I've run out of calories and I'm borrowing from the next day. I am disappointed in myself. I am angry at myself. I am so angry at myself! Why can't I do this??? Why do I get up every single day and just **eat too much**? I feel like a failure to myself and everything I stand for."

I was exhausted, frustrated, angry and lost. I can hardly re-read that entry without feeling that deep pit start to open up and pull me in. And while that was one of my more colorful rants... it certainly wasn't too far off base from how I felt about myself *most of the time* for close to a decade.

And I had *lost* the weight.

And I exercised, daily.

And I was a personal trainer and a weight loss coach.

I know I'm not alone. When I read those words, I know that I am not the only person who has felt that way because I've heard those very same words in the voices of my friends, my clients, my family members, strangers whose blogs I've read, contestants on TV shows. In working with hundreds of people trying to lose weight, I have found that my second journal entry is how many people feel when they try to lose weight.

Carrying extra weight is not just a physical burden. When you're overweight, you carry that baggage mentally. It can become the lens through which you see the world, the perspective that colors your experiences. Being overweight can keep you from participating fully in your life. Without question being overweight affects your physical health, but it also affects your mental and emotional state. It can keep you from seeing yourself as a whole person and give you a reason to put off life experiences, with the thought "I'll do that when I lose the weight...."

Rachel was one of my first clients who I was able to coach through a similar transformation, and it was with her that I first recognized that this process was one that could be taught and shared with others in order to improve their weight loss success. I began working with Rachel on the basics of weight loss, focusing first on using a calorie budget and making choices that would keep her feeling healthy and energetic all day long. Over the course of a year of us working together, Rachel lost 40 pounds. As her coach, I was thrilled with her progress, but Rachel had over 50 pounds left that she wanted to lose, and she felt stuck.

At 58 years old, Rachel had struggled with her weight for her entire life. She couldn't even remember a time when she felt happy with her weight. It was clear to me that Rachel completely identified herself as an overweight woman. In fact, her imagination would barely allow her to visualize what life might be like at her healthy goal weight. One day, after she had been at her new weight for nearly six months, I asked her if she could close her eyes and visualize herself at her goal weight. She couldn't.

Since her goal weight was 50 pounds away, I asked her if she could imagine herself 25 pounds less. She shook her head no.

20 pounds? Another head shake.

15 pounds? Still no.

10 pounds? Slowly, Rachel nodded. "Yes," she said, "I can imagine myself weighing ten pounds less than I do now."

"Well," I asked her, "how about eleven pounds?"

We finally determined that Rachel could imagine herself weighing about 12 pounds less than her current weight, but anything past that was just a big, blank unknown in her mind. I asked her why she thought she was unable to imagine herself at her goal weight. She said she didn't know, but I was pretty sure she did, so I kept pressing her.

"Fear?" she finally said, with a note of hesitation and doubt in her voice.

"Yes," I replied. "But fear of what?"

She was quiet while she thought about it for a long time. "Fear of failure," she finally admitted, quietly. It was an admission to herself, not to me.

Rachel, who for more than 50 years had only thought of herself as an overweight woman, was afraid to move forward for fear that she'd fail. That that failure would lead to disappointment, guilt, shame – all these emotions that we work hard to avoid. I gave Rachel an analogy to help demonstrate to her why it was so hard for her to move past her programmed fear.

"Imagine you came to me and wanted me to help you train for marathon." This is a task that I would venture to say might possibly be easier than a 90 pound weight loss journey! But, a task Rachel could hardly imagine herself doing nonetheless. "Now let's say we had just completed our 2-mile run. And it was really, really hard – as a 2 mile run would probably be for any first time runner. If you thought about that 2 mile run and thought, *"if 2 miles felt like that, I'll never be able to 26 miles!"*, then of course, of course, you would quit the training.

If you recognize that 26 miles would come only after 2 miles was mastered, then 2.2 miles, then 2.4 miles, then 3 miles and so on, you would progress forward in your marathon training. However, when someone faces an overwhelming task that they can't even visualize themselves completing even the first step can trigger fear.

The light bulb was on for Rachel but the question remained. "How do I move past that fear?" I just smiled, because that was the question I had been hoping she would ask.

The desire to move past fear and to make the shift away from this negative, self-deprecating way of thinking is the missing piece for weight loss. It's where most "diet plans" fall short. It's where most people get stuck. It's where I've helped my clients move forward, and where I can help you.

My change in thinking about my body and my weight came about almost by accident. I had enrolled in coaching training and as part of our program we were provided with a coach to work with us once a week on whatever we wanted. I was fortunate enough to be assigned to a coach who had started his own successful consulting/coaching practice, and I wanted him to coach me on the challenges I faced trying to launch my own business. In just a few sessions, he helped me identify some of my fears about having to market my own skills and some of the limiting beliefs I had about what kind of success I could achieve. He helped me listen to the way I was talking to myself about business, money, sales, and my own skills. As I changed my internal dialogue, and ultimately my beliefs, launching my business came more naturally.

One day, I found myself wondering if the act of changing my thinking, which had helped me change my approach to launching my business, could have a similar effect on my body and my weight. I was so fed up with my current approach, the vicious cycle of be in control, lapse, beat myself up, attempt to rein myself in again. I was willing to try anything, so I decided to dive in with this approach focused on changing my thoughts about my body.

It was about 3 months later that I found myself writing that journal entry on my way back from Christmas vacation, suspended in the clouds, feeling an overwhelming mixture of disbelief and gratitude. I immediately began using these strategies with the people I worked with and started seeing the amazing results for them as well.

I wanted to write this book in order to create something that anyone could pick up, easily read through and then immediately start using. I want to help people climb out of the pit of frustration, sadness and discontentment that the struggle of losing weight often creates. I call this process Inside Out Weight Management, because it addresses the way your core beliefs and internal dialogue affect the choices you make every day that determine whether or not you'll lose weight.

This book is intended for people who have acquired the basic "how to" knowledge of losing weight, and especially those who have tried diet after diet, and find themselves unable to sustain their momentum for more than a few months, or few weeks, or even a few days at a time. It is even for those who have lost weight and who are trying to maintain it, but who find that it's a daily personal struggle. The most common thing I hear from my clients when they are starting out is that they know *how* to lose weight... but that knowledge has simply not been enough. Something else has been missing. This is the missing piece.

This book is different from most "diet books" because it's *not* a diet book. I'm not here to tell you <u>how</u> to lose weight – there are plenty of other experts out there who do such an exceptional job with that. Unfortunately, there are plenty of others out there who do more harm than good with the diet plans they promote – and the result of using some of those unrealistic weight loss plans is the negative programming many people who have tried and failed to maintain weight loss have today.

I am not going to tell you how to lose weight, but I am going to explain to you why it has been a struggle for you to lose or to maintain a weight loss. More importantly though, I am going to walk you through the steps that will help you coach yourself through the challenges that have made weight loss hard for you in the past.

The end result of using Inside Out Weight Management is that you should feel that it's easier to get and stay motivated for weight loss. You will also feel more positive and optimistic about weight loss and you should find the behaviors for weight loss easier to sustain.

I will also spend a large portion of this book explaining what emotional eating is and how to break free from the hurtful cycle of habitual, uncontrolled eating. Whether it is ice cream or almonds, a healthy relationship with food means that you're in control when you choose how much, how often and what you eat. Using this program can help you establish and maintain that control.

My approach to creating sustainable weight loss from the inside out has two steps. The first step is examining and changing your weight loss programming. The second is tackling emotional eating. Many of the ideas introduced in the first section of the book about changing your weight loss programming will support the ideas explained in the second part on emotional eating, so I would encourage you to read both parts. These two steps are the essential piece to creating the healthy lifestyle you deserve.

The process can also be used to create motivation and forward momentum in any other area of your life where you feel stuck. Using the same principles that I've laid out in my Inside Out Weight Management program my clients have made changes in their careers, improved their finances and created more engaging relationships. The process of change is the same no matter what area of your life you want to apply it to. The steps are not difficult to master, though they require daily practice once understood.

While the idea of a new process you have to do every day may sound overwhelming, think about this: many years ago, someone introduced you to a new practice that done once or twice a day, would improve your health and make you feel better. You probably didn't know how to do this thing when it was first demonstrated to you, and in fact you probably required some prompting, reminding, and maybe even bribing to consistently practice this behavior once or twice a day. Once mastered, almost everyone I know does this behavior, without thinking, each and every day and night. They recognize its long term benefits, and the practice itself has come habitual.

The steps of Inside Out Weight Management are as easy to master as brushing your teeth. The ultimate objective of this program is that the practice of reprogramming will become as automatic and habitual as every American's twice-a-day teeth brushing ritual. And while I can't promise that Inside Out Weight Management will leave you cavity free, it will benefit your life in ways you may not even be able to close your eyes and imagine right now.

Part I: Inside Out Weight Management

Chapter 2: What is Programming?

Remember the first time you drove a car? You had a lot to think about: where to put your hands, how often to look in the rear view mirror, how the car should line up with the side of the road, and how far away you should be from the car in front of you. Chances are you didn't even have the radio on! How much of your attention did you have to devote to driving that car when you first learned?

Most people (thankfully) answer that they gave almost 100% of their attention to learning to drive. Now, when I ask my next question: "how much attention do you give to driving your car today?" the answer varies. It's usually met with nervous laughter, looks around the room and guilty shrugs. But the truth is, almost all of us pay less than 100% attention to driving our car today because we have set *programming* around what it means to drive a car. Everything we heard, learned, read, and experienced about driving a car has been filed away in a set of "programmed thoughts." Those thoughts are subconsciously accessed every time we put the key in the ignition.

Programming doesn't require a great deal of conscious thought to work. If you've ever pulled in your driveway and realized you don't really remember the ride home, but you must have taken the right turns, then you have experienced subconscious programming.

Our programming can change as our experiences changes. Maybe you drive down a back country road to your house and you're used to going 10 or 20 miles over the speed limit. One day, a cop pulls out behind you, lights flashing.

Chances are, your programming around driving down that road is going to change. Depending on how getting a ticket impacted you, the change may be permanent or temporary.

I got my first speeding ticket just one year after I got my driver's license. I was headed over to a friend's house and was coming down a hill on a suburban road when I got clocked doing 47 in a 35. I was *so* upset to get my first ticket and sobbed into the payphone back at school when I called my Dad to tell him. I don't remember much about what happened afterwards, except that I had to babysit for a few Saturdays in a row to "barter" the cost of the lawyer fee (my father's friend) who represented me in traffic court. It turned out to be a small price to pay for the lesson but I can assure you it did little to damper my lead foot.

I was fortunate enough to go the next 13 years without a speeding ticket, until one day while headed over to a friend's house to walk our dogs I saw those awful flashing lights in my rearview mirror and felt my stomach sink. I knew I had been speeding and was not likely to get off with a warning. The motorcycle cop barely exchanged any words with me except to ask for my license and registration and to return with my ticket. This time, I felt the impact. The lawyer fee came out of my own pocket, and I was confronted with the consequence of my ticket every time I paid my car insurance. The increase wasn't substantial but it was an obvious enough reminder to me each month that I can now call myself a reformed speeder. I keep the cruise control on about 7 over the limit at almost all times and I do my best to ignore the jerks that zoom up behind me and gave me dagger looks for maintaining my speed. (And I know that I very well may have been one of those jerks not too long ago.)

Whether behavior change is permanent or temporary often depends on how strongly the experience of what we've been through impacts us. And it's nearly impossible to predict what types of experiences will change someone's programming. We all have loved ones who have suffered a major health crisis, such as a heart attack or the diagnosis of diabetes, and think surely it will be a wake up call to get them to change their behaviors – and it isn't. Or, sometimes it is a seemingly innocuous moment – the sight of an unflattering photograph, reading a magazine article, a passing comment from a stranger – that becomes the impetus for change. It's impossible to know what moment will be the catalyst for long-term change, because it's completely dependent on each person's past programming.

Programming is a collection of thoughts that your subconscious has gathered and stored away, to be accessed whenever you start thinking about or engaging in a certain set of circumstances. Your programming is based on what you've heard, seen or lived through around that specific experience. It's my belief that programming allows us to store away "old" information as a set group of thoughts, feelings and actions in order to allow our conscious self to focus on developing new skills or go through new experiences.

Each of us has a set of programming around weight loss, body image and the actions that correlate with a healthy lifestyle, such as exercise or making healthy food decisions. Every time you think about weight loss, you subconsciously access this past programming. The emotions that this past programming generates are what determine whether or not the actions that support weight loss will be easy to follow through on.

Some of the programming that I have heard from myself or my clients sounds like this:

- I'm big boned.

- I'm a stress eater.

- I'm just addicted to sugar.

- Eating healthy is so boring.

- I HATE exercise.

- My whole family is overweight – so I'm just doomed to be overweight too.

- I *have* to have my pasta... I couldn't live without it.

- I have a slow metabolism.

- Why bother? I'll just regain it.

Sometimes this programming is spoken outright. Other times it is implied through other statements. "Why bother," is often implied by, "Well, I messed up today... I'll start tomorrow!"

Sometimes programming originates in our childhood, when we are most impressionable. I work with many people who grew up hearing the infamous line, "Finish what's on your plate! There's starving children...." You can imagine how the act of leaving behind food on your plate (or "wasting food" as I usually hear it referred to) goes *against* one's subconscious programming if this was a phrase that was repeated day in and day out at dinner time.

In my classes, we would discuss many different strategies for weight loss. Every year when we discussed the challenges of holiday cooking and hosting parties, someone would inevitably mention the problem of leftovers. I'd ask the group what they could do with leftovers after the holiday was over. Suggestions included sending it home with guests, freezing it, taking it into the office or giving it to a neighbor.

I would stand there waiting. "One other option exists," I'd say, knowing the reaction that was coming. They would look around at each other, confused, and try to think of what option I was referring to.

"You could *throw it out.*"

Chaos would erupt. The idea of throwing out food, for many people, feels reckless and wasteful. And I agree it may not be the best option as far as reducing waste or being economical. But it *is* an option. We are so programmed not to waste food that even when there's a possibility that keeping that food in our home could sabotage our health goals, we still can't bear to throw it out.

I know many other people who were told to "Finish what's on your plate and then you can have dessert." Well, what does that teach us about what's on our plate? That we must suffer through broccoli to get to brownies!?

Programming is deeply rooted in the messages we heard growing up. These messages might be about food, such as the above example, but they were also about body image and weight. Sometimes the messages aren't clearly related to weight loss, but in my clients' lives they show up there.

For example, recently I worked with a woman named Sarah who has been doing a lot of work to understand her past programming. She realized today that the message she heard growing up was that while her parents would always love her unconditionally, other people's love would be conditional and would depend on her behaviors and her appearance. Her people pleasing behavior has spilled over into her grown up life, and she felt a discrepancy between her past programming and her desire to take action with healthy food choices whenever she felt that those choices might inconvenience someone else, like her husband or friends.

Past programming doesn't just stop in childhood. A great deal of programming is created as soon as someone enters the world of diets. In fact, the word "diet" itself has a whole set of programming for most people! And usually, not a good one.

When I ask people what feelings the word "diet" brings up for them, I usually hear words like "guilt," "frustration," "deprivation," "misery" – even "anger." No one has ever once said anything remotely warm and fuzzy about the word diet. Although we may want and feel good about the results from a diet, the act of dieting itself rarely makes people feel good.

Past diets that have created feelings of deprivation, guilt and failed attempts or regained weight can generate some really powerful programming around "weight loss" in general. If your past programming includes a lot of disappointment, frustration, and guilt, then it's no wonder that you find it hard to sustain the behaviors needed to create weight loss. Merely thinking about these behaviors taps into the emotions tied to the programming.

How long do you think you are going to do something that makes you feel frustrated, guilty, disappointed, even resentful or overwhelmed?

Not very long.

When I ask this question in my group, the light bulb goes on for many people who have wondered why they just can't seem to stick with a weight loss plan even when they know exactly what to do and want to lose weight. Struggling to sustain weight loss behaviors is very common, and has nothing to do with willpower or education. It almost always has to do with the conflict between those behaviors and the emotions they generate. It will take a *monumental* amount of effort to do something for a long time that makes you feel awful.

Once I discovered that programming was the key to sustaining long term behaviors, I started doing some "research" into what my own programming might be. It wasn't very hard research – all I had to do was read some of those journal entries or listen to my rambling inner monologue anytime I stepped on a scale, put on a pair of pants, stood in front of the pantry or contemplated going for a run.

The first thing I heard loud and clear in my own programming was that I felt like I had to be perfect. I was a personal trainer and a weight loss coach – <u>I had to be perfect</u>. I feared that if I couldn't be perfect, how could the people that I tried to help ever take me seriously? Consequently, any time I partook in any "less than perfect" behavior – an exercise routine skipped, a 2nd piece of dessert – I felt like a complete failure. It became a vicious cycle – striving for perfection, failing and beating myself up. I constantly felt guilty and inadequate.

I also realized that a big piece of my programming was the belief that I was a stress eater. This was something I not only told myself, I told others. This wasn't merely a subconscious piece of programming; I was willing to broadcast this piece of programming to the world! I thought that this was just part of who I was, and that I might as well confess to it. Since misery loves company, I also found that referring to myself as a stress eater was a way to relate to other people and share a common bond. This bond with people just further reinforced my label, without me even realizing it.

Why was this so damaging? This hurtful behavior has been explained in many different languages, from the Bible to Buddha to Descartes. I like Buddha's version, because it is succinct and to the point.

"We are what we think."

Programming is so powerful, not only for the emotions it generates, but for what I call "data collection." When you declare, to yourself or to others, to be a certain thing, you begin to collect evidence to support this statement. Who doesn't like to be right? If you declare yourself to be a stress eater, a stress eater you shall be.

Our identity is, at its simplest form, a collection of stories we tell ourselves about ourselves. Sometimes these stories come from things we've heard from other people or the way we've explained certain experiences we've had. They often begin in childhood and the longer we've been telling a particular story, the more it feels like a fact.

As I declared to myself and to others that I was a stress eater – Wheat Thins being my usual vice – I collected evidence to prove this was the truth. I noticed every time that I felt that my willpower to resist the goods of the pantry started to give. My thesis writing sessions could have been sponsored by Nabisco I bought so many of those darn yellow boxes! I scolded myself as I added up the calories in my food log. I would say to myself, elbow deep in a bag of Tostitos, "you are ruining the great workout you just had!" But, I had declared myself a stress eater, and a stress eater I was. I felt powerless to stop.

I never understood how powerful my own declaration was, and how simply declaring it over and over again reinforced the very behavior I wanted so badly to diminish.

When you declare yourself to be something, you naturally will take part in the behaviors that will make it true. A cycle is born when our behaviors then reinforce that identify, and we become even more firmly entrenched in the idea of who we are. I like to say each of us has a story we tell about ourselves, and then we look for the moments in our life that make that story our reality. Being a stress eater was party of my story, and I paid great attention to the times when I was eating in response to stress.

It never occurred to me that I was the author of my story and just as I had created one reality, I could create a new one.

Rachel's weight loss was also affected by her programming. One day, during a session with Rachel, I asked her how long she had felt like she was overweight. She said she could remember being about four or five years old, sitting in school thinking about how tight her skirt felt.

Rachel had over 50 years of programming that told her she *was* fat! This was the story she continued to tell herself, even as she was trying to change. She struggled to maintain the changes in her behaviors, and I quickly understood that her past programming – 50 years of past programming – were not supporting the changes she was trying to make.

As long as she continued to think of herself as a fat person, she would "collect the data" that supported this. She took note every time she ate a portion that was too big, every time she made a higher calorie choice and every day she skipped exercise. Rachel had a hard time congratulating herself on the healthy choices she made, because her past programming had caused her to pay attention to the behaviors that supported "I am fat."

Rachel was understandably overwhelmed when I began explaining programming to her. She was at first resistant to the idea that she would have to begin changing her story – thinking of herself as a healthy or fit person – before the behavior changes would come easily to her.

"But how can I think of myself as I thin person when I look in the mirror and I see a fat person?" she asked me. She was clearly exasperated by the challenge I was posing to her.

Everyone faces this same challenge when they start reprogramming. How can you tell yourself you are one thing, when the physical evidence indicates something else? We often feel like we owe it to ourselves to be "realistic" and state the facts about our life. For many, reprogramming feels like denial and they fear the situation will just get worse. I understand this, and I felt that way myself. I was afraid that letting go would result in me going out of control. But I was also tired of trying the same things over and over again, and getting the same results. I felt like I had nothing to to lose by trying something new. If you are ready to admit that the strategies you have tried in the past have not worked, then you will be ready to try reprogramming.

Reprogramming is an act of intention. It requires responding to your automatic thoughts, which can be difficult. If you wake up in the morning and stub your toe, what's the first thing you think?

Most people's response is usually "ouch!!" or some other four letter word. Sometimes we go so far as to think, "Great – this day is already off to a bad start." And sure enough, the day goes downhill from there. The traffic is jammed, your coffee spills, the meeting runs over, someone gives you bad customer service ... the list goes on.

In that moment, when you stub your toe, you have an automatic thought about that experience. The rest of the day, you may even continue to pay attention to the facts that support the idea that you just got up on the wrong side of the bed that day. However, if you were able to pause for second and react to your automatic thought you might end up changing the course of the entire day!

"GAHHHH, AGGGH, OUCH."

"Now wait a second... did that really hurt? No. *I am fine.*"

And on you go. Imagine if you will, that you woke up every morning and stubbed your toe. If you practiced your new "I am fine" statement immediately upon stubbing your toe every morning, what do you think would eventually happen?

(I know, I know. You'd just move your nightstand. Seriously, why did you put it right there in the first place?)

Eventually, upon stubbing your toe you would automatically think, "I am fine." Stubbing your toe would become a non-event, something that barely registered on your radar screen.

Did you ever notice how people who have healthy relationships with food don't get flipped out over eating a huge meal every once in awhile? It's as much of a non-event as a toe stub to them, due to their programming. For many people who are trying to lose weight, overeating at one meal leads to a chain reaction of automatic thoughts starting with "I blew it," followed by "I have no control" and then often finishing up with "I might as well wait until tomorrow to get back on track." The automatic reaction to overeating is as programmed as the reaction to stubbing your toe.

Using intentional thinking to replace automatic thoughts helps us create new programming. New behaviors are then much easier when you have a different set of automatic thoughts. This is why I call this process Inside Out Weight Management. Although the long term goal is to change our behaviors, we have to start from the inside out and change our thoughts first.

For Rachel, for myself and countless others, the thoughts we have about our weight, our food choices, our bodies and ourselves are as automatic as a reaction to stubbing your toe in the morning. Practiced over and over again for years, they've become so deeply entrenched in the subconscious that they shape our reality.

Chapter 3: Step One: Recognize Your Programming

In order to change your programming, we need to understand why some programming helps us and some programming hurts us. As my client Rachel found out, the key to long term success in any change process comes from the inside out: from changing the *thoughts* in order to change the behaviors.

Every action we take depends on how we're feeling in the exact moment we make a decision.

French fries or salad? Depends on how you feel.

Run or sit on the couch? Depends on how you feel.

Go to bed early or stay up late?

Keep your lunch date with a friend or cancel last minute?

Finish the report for work or check email for the fifteenth time?

Every action we take depends on how we feel in the moment we make the choice about what to do. And our feelings come from a very specific place: our thoughts.

This is called the "The TFA Chain." The "TFA Chain" stands for thoughts, feelings and actions. The theory states that your thoughts create your feelings and then feelings create action. When it comes to making change, most people start with their actions without realizing that these actions stem from feelings and thoughts. The TFA Chain, in my experience, is one of the most simple principles for understanding part of human motivation, decision and choices. It helps us understand why behavior change is so difficult and more importantly, how to make change both easier and permanent.

The TFA Chain is not new, and not something I have created. It has been around for years and has been documented for use in everything from working with alcoholism to marriage counseling to starting a business. While the origin source is unknown, the idea that "thoughts create feelings and feelings create action" is identified by Dr. Robert Perkinson, PhD in his handbook Chemical Dependency Counseling: A Practical Guide.[1] Dr. Perkinson's use of TFA is developed from the larger framework called "Situations, Thoughts, Consequences" that was developed by Richard Nelson-Jones and explained in his book Practical Counselling and and Helping Skills.[2]

When we try to create change, we usually start with actions. We try to change our behaviors. We set goals that are specific and measureable and action-oriented. Goal-setting is a valuable skill and definitely a part of behavior change. But when we fall short of our goals, we get frustrated and blame ourselves. We chalk it up to busy schedules, lack of willpower, or bad timing. We blame ourselves, we feel guilty, we give up.

If you've tried losing weight before and not been successful, or lost and regained it, your subconscious thoughts about weight loss might be something like: "I can't do it. Weight loss is hard." Or "I might lose, but I'll probably regain."

You're not consciously thinking these thoughts as you set off on your weight loss journey, loading up your grocery cart with baby carrots and apples, signing up for that gym membership with optimism and hope, sneaking that pair of skinny jeans out of your closet and dreaming of the day they'll go past your mid-thigh. The "I can't do it" thought is buried down deep – it's buried beneath the initial excitement, hope and optimism that accompany the fresh start of a new weight loss journey. But it's there.

For many people, "I can't do it" is a stronger thought than "I can do it." If history creates programming, then the past tried-and-failed efforts have generated a programming around failure.

"I can't" or "I must be perfect" or "I don't have the willpower" or "It's going to be so hard" or whatever the past programming might be creates a multitude of emotions – none of them very warm and fuzzy. Worry. Deprivation. Guilt. Apathy. Frustration. Anger. *Fear.*

If the thought of weight loss generated any of those negative feelings, how long do you think you would continue to take actions in the name of weight loss?

As I've said before, probably not very long. This is where most people feel that internal struggle to maintain weight loss behaviors.

For me, every time I "acted" in the name of weight loss, I brought up the programming "I must be perfect!" Every time I got out my food log, packed a gym bag, or grocery shopped, I'd trigger that programming. Sometimes I was conscious of this thought, but often I wasn't. Regardless of my awareness of this thought, it made me <u>feel</u> stressed, overwhelmed and really angry. I'd make progress for a few days, sometimes even a few weeks, and then I'd fall off the wagon and wonder why I just couldn't do it.

Negative programming is pervasive in weight loss. Few people have positive programming around weight loss. My clients who have found weight loss to be the easiest are often the ones who have never tried to lose weight before. Their programming around weight loss is minimal, and their thoughts tend to be predominately more positive and hopeful. Those strong emotions of hope, optimism and confidence make the actions that create weight loss much easier and sustainable.

Becoming aware of your programming is the first step in creating weight loss from the inside out. Begin by listening to the stories you tell yourself about weight loss, about food, about exercise and about what it means to be healthy. Begin by listening to the stories you tell yourself about *who you are*.

When I begin this step with a client, I often ask them to keep a small notebook and to jot down any internal dialogue they have with themselves that they think might be relevant. Other clients have sent themselves an email every time they hear a relevant thought and others have kept an index card in a pocket or in their wallets.

Capturing your programming is critical, even if it may feel a little bit tedious or even silly. It will allow you to look for reoccurring themes, and the thoughts that are generating the most powerful emotions for you. This will allow you to make the most meaningful changes possible.

This step was fairly easy for me, as I had almost 10 years of journals to reflect back on! I found that I talked about my body, my weight and food in my journals all the time. The first thing that got me excited about making changes was wondering what I was going to be able to do with all that extra brain power once I wasn't thinking about my weight all the time!

If you're ready to begin this powerful change process, this is the first step. Create **awareness** around your programming. Spend as long as you need on this first step, until you feel that you have sufficiently captured the "reoccurring themes" in your programming.

If you need help getting started, spend some time thinking about what you learned as a child when it came to food, to weight, even about yourself. What messages did you hear from your parents, from other adults, from your friends?

Was food used as a reward or associated with a very positive experience? Was anyone important in your life – a parent, family member, a friend – always concerned about or talking about their weight? Were foods labeled as "good" and "bad"?

Reflect, too, on what sort of things you saw people in your life doing. Did you know anyone who was on a diet when you were little? How did the adults in your life treat food when they were growing up? How did they treat themselves? Try to capture as many details as you can during this step. Some of these details may not be obvious or easy at first, but if you remain open to the idea of reflecting you might be surprised at what memories return to you.

Casey, a client of mine who claimed she could eat a half bag of Hershey kisses in a night, experienced a turning point in her weight loss efforts with this exercise. After going through this exercise, she suddenly remembered that when she was a little girl her mom would keep a stash of chocolate hidden in the laundry room. When her mom was upset about something, she'd see her go to the laundry room and take a piece of chocolate. "Don't tell Daddy," she'd say. Occasionally she would add something like, "Chocolate is therapy for women," or would slip her a piece saying, "Just between you and me!"

Casey had a love affair with chocolate all her life and often turned to sweets in times of stress, but hid this from her boyfriend. She felt guilty as her boyfriend was trying to help her lose weight, and she couldn't understand why she felt so embarrassed to tell him about her secret chocolate habit. The answer became clear when she recalled this memory – something she hadn't thought about for years. Her mom had modeled the behavior of using chocolate as an antidote to stress, and her words had implied it was something that men wouldn't understand. In fact, by including her daughter in the complicit act of eating chocolate, it actually became a very special ritual for my client. It was no wonder she felt such joy as she unwrapped the foil around a Hershey kiss. The sight of the milk chocolate inside was transporting her back to a special secret shared between her and her mother!

Andrew, another client of mine, had a hard time figuring out what his programming had been. Both of his parents had been normal weight, and he didn't really remember them making a lot of fuss about diets, or even having to finish his plate. Andrew's weight issues begin in his late 30s, and his biggest challenge was that he loved to eat out. One day, it occurred to me to ask Andrew how often his family ate out when he was growing up.

"Rarely," he told me. "Special occasions - maybe our birthdays, but never really more than that." Andrew had come from a large family, and though his parents never talked about money, he had always known not to ask for too much or that there wasn't a lot of extra money for indulgences. He eventually came to realize that he loved to go out to eat now simply because *he could* - a luxury that wasn't afforded in childhood that he could indulge in as much as he wanted to now as a grown-up. Andrew's past programming was focused on there being "not enough" and this created feelings of deprivation and disappointment. Whenever Andrew tried to lose weight, and he told himself he shouldn't go out to eat as much, it sparked those emotions of deprivation that were programmed from his childhood.

Our programming is not always about food or our bodies, though. As I mentioned, my own programming was around trying to be perfect. However, this had little to do with any messages I heard or behaviors I saw modeled around food. I was a good student growing up, and I excelled in school. I thrived off the praise that I got from teachers and parents, and even my friends. I am thankful that I had this programming, because my desire to push myself to be the best I could be meant I was able to go to some excellent schools and have wonderful life experiences because of that. However, while this programming was beneficial for me in one aspect of my life it clearly did not serve me well when it came to my body and my food choices.

This is also a good example of how programming is not necessarily negative or positive. Your programming may have served you very well in one area of your life, even if it's created challenges or issues for you in another area of your life. If your programming is around being a caretaker for others, this may be something you take great pride in. Others acknowledge you for being generous and compassionate. This is, of course, a very positive trait in many aspects of life. However, if it has created a situation where you have a hard time putting that programming aside to take care of yourself, it can become a detriment as much as it is an asset.

Each of us has a story with many chapters that have shaped and molded our programming around food and our bodies. The only way to make long lasting changes is to become crystal clear about what that story is, and what you want it to be. Pay attention to the way you talk to yourself about food or your body. Listen to your internal dialogue; take note of your beliefs, journal how you feel about yourself and your choices. You may even want to ask someone you trust what types of things they have heard you say about yourself, about your body, about food or exercise or health. Sometimes those around us are even more tuned in to what we're saying about ourselves than we may be.

You cannot skip this step, as hard as it may be. You have to become absolutely clear on what your programming is if you would like to change it. This step may take you no more than a few hours, or it may take you a few weeks. Take your time and try to gather as much information as possible. I would recommend writing down what you've come up with in order to make the next step, changing your programming, easier.

Chapter 4: Step Two: Rewriting Your Story

If you completed the step from the chapter before, you should be crystal clear about your programming. In the last chapter, I introduced you to the TFA Chain. The TFA chain explains that thoughts create feelings, and feelings create action. Every action we take – from choosing what to have for dinner, to deciding to take a walk, to staying up too late – is rooted in how we are feeling in the moment we make that decision. How we feel comes directly from what we are thinking in that moment.

Programming is automatic thinking. Just like the "owwww!!!" reaction when you stub your toe, your programming is playing in the background of your subconscious whether or not you pay attention to it. Your programming is generating certain types of emotions that are going to determine whether or not you'll sustain the actions you say you want to take to create a healthy life. If that programming creates emotions like frustration, worry, disgust, guilt, apathy or fear, you are going to find that taking action that supports a healthy lifestyle is going to be quite challenging and hard to sustain.

Think about the beginning of all weight loss plans. Our thoughts are focused on our impending success. As we eagerly anticipate the delight in seeing the scale move, the loose feeling of our clothing, the rush of working out at the gym, we are filled with feelings of hopefulness, confidence and motivation. It is easy to make changes. "Why, of COURSE, I'll have the grilled chicken," we think gleefully.

Fast forward to a few weeks later. Or maybe even a few days later. The scale has been slower than we hoped. The gym? Do you know you have to *sweat* when you go there? Our clothes fit the same. Our thoughts become focused on the stagnation. On what is *not* happening. We begin to feel discouraged and frustrated. It becomes easier to drive straight home rather than to the gym. "Just one more cookie won't hurt," begins to become a daily mantra.

Soon, the scale is moving in the other direction. The gym membership is being autodrafted, each month a daily reminder of the money we're wasting. The pants? We're buying a bigger size. Now our thoughts are totally focused on failure. The emotions that accompany this are guilt, disappointment, and worry that we're right back where we started. "What's the point," we think as we order the onion rings instead of the fruit salad.

And thus, the slippery cycle of weight loss. Most of us are accustomed to looking at the actions of this cycle to determine where to make changes. Maybe it was the wrong diet book I bought! Maybe I needed to hire a personal trainer! Maybe I need one of those fancy digital scales that tells me how hydrated I am! **We eternally tinker with the endpoints and wonder why each time we end up back at the place we started.**

If we were to move backwards through the TFA chain, we would arrive at the most powerful point of change:

41

our thoughts. The actions we take originate with our feelings. Our feelings are determined by our thoughts. Changing action requires working backwards through the chain to examine, and ultimately change, our thoughts.

What emotions would you need to be feeling in order to easily and automatically sustain the type of actions that support a healthy lifestyle? Most people agree that they need to be feeling positive emotions. Confidence, optimism, competence, hope, excitement.... All of these are examples of emotions that instill in us the desire to move forward easily with actions that sustain a healthy lifestyle. These are the same emotions we often experience in the beginning of our weight loss efforts that make healthy choices seem to happen naturally.

Emotions are a reaction to our thoughts. Our thoughts are really just the story we tell ourselves about a situation, and it's up to us to determine what we want that story to be. Remember the toe stub? Thoughts often feel automatic and out of our control, but if we can recognize a thought that is generating a negative emotion we can react to it and choose a new thought. Over time, your subconscious would automatically begin to accept that new thought as automatic. This is why recognizing your programming is the first step in the process of change.

Everyone's weight varies from one day to the next, based on fluid retention. That day to day fluctuation is totally normal, but there are a variety of different reactions to those fluctuations from one person to the next. This is one example of how a specific situation can generate automatic thoughts, even though there are other stories that are equally as plausible.

Let's take a specific example. Sydney, a client of mine, weighs every single day despite my suggestion that that may not be helpful for her.

On Monday morning, Sydney steps on the scale before showering and sees that she weighs 237 pounds. She is delighted. This is a 20 pound weight loss for her, which was her first milestone. She sends me an email, and I celebrate this fact with her as well.

Monday's a typical day for Sydney, who is an account manager for a large retail company. She sits at her desk most of the day, goes for a walk after work and goes out to an Italian restaurant with her husband for a late dinner. She is proud of herself for her weight loss, and orders the soup and salad, basking in her good choices.

The next morning, Sydney steps on the scale. She is in shock to see she now weighs 241 pounds. In fact, she steps on the scale three more times to make sure she was not mistaken. Instantly, she feels deflated. She feels like a failure and is embarrassed for bragging that she had met her goal. All day long, she is thinking about that weight and is so disappointed that she came so close to her goal and lost it. Her lunch choices are poor, and at the end of the day, she drives right past the gym. By the time I saw her two days later, her official weight on my scale was 2 pounds up from our last weigh in. She knew she was off track but admitted to not really feeling like getting on track.

Sydney's story may sound dramatic to you, or you may be nodding your head in understanding. Sydney's reaction is not unusual – not for Sydney, as she experiences these ups and downs on a weekly basis – and not for a number of the people I have worked with whose emotional ups and downs can be totally dictated by 3 digital numbers.

Sydney had an opportunity to tell herself a number of different stories about that number she saw on Tuesday. The story she told herself was based on her past programming. Having tried to lose weight a number of times in the past, Sydney's past programming subconsciously told her she had failed again and that losing weight was going to be very hard. While Sydney might initially have a hard time feeling any other way than upset and disappointed in response to an uptick on the scale, just like stubbing her toe, she has a chance to *react* to that automatic thought and choose a new thought.

Reflecting on her day before, Sydney could have considered what factors really create day to day fluctuations in weight. For instance, Sydney's soup and salad combo at the Italian restaurant, while potentially lower in calories that the Spaghetti Bolognese, were probably quite high in salt. This extra sodium her body was processing probably resulted in some fluid retention. How might Sydney feel differently if her interpretation of the 4 pound uptick was "Hmm. Well I couldn't possibly have eaten an extra 14,000 calories to *really* gain 4 pounds.... It must be water weight."

Poor Sydney. She ran around all day on Tuesday beating herself up for failing, eating her co-worker's secret stash of chocolate at lunch and standing up her date with the Stair Mill, all because she assumed she had really gained 4 pounds, a feat that would have required an extra 14,000 calories. It's kind of silly isn't it? Almost as silly as allowing ourselves to have a bad day, because we got out of bed a little too close to our nightstand. Yet we do it...all the time!

Sydney's automatic interpretation of the event is difficult to change, but her reaction to that automatic thought would generate new emotions. She might feel relieved, still hopeful and even more determined to move forward and keep that 20 pound milestone in place (or pass it!), by accepting that she made great choices the day before and may simply be retaining water.

This is just one example of how automatic programming can shape our perception of our event and generate very powerful emotions that determine what actions you will take moving forward. There's a really easy to way to tell whether or not the story you're telling yourself about an event is going to support healthy actions.

Feeling bad? Stressed? Anxious? Frustrated? Change your thoughts. Your feelings are a barometer that can be used to help you recognize moments when you would want to change your thoughts.

The only person who can determine *what* you think is YOU. This can be a tough concept for people to accept. So much of our programming is automatic in order to allow us to get through the day with all the many tasks we have to accomplish and master. I'm not asking you to change every single thought you have, or even to monitor every single thought you have. Just monitor how you're feeling, and when you're feeling any type of low, negative emotion that's a sign that you need to tune in to what thought you're having and make a choice to change it.

This step involves a little bit of "fake it til you make it." The first time Sydney tells herself "it's just water weight," she will probably still feel a little bit of disbelief, and accompanying that, the residual guilt, disappointment and frustration that her automatic programming generated. The more often she practices reacting to that situation with her new, intentional thought, the stronger that thought will become, eventually permeating the subconscious and replacing the old automatic thoughts.

Often times, I find people worry that if they change their thoughts that they're going to get off track. There is this really strong fear among those who have tried to lose weight that if they are kind, forgiving and loving towards themselves that they are just going to go crazy and eat anything and everything and get wildly out of control. They feel really strongly that the "reality check" of making themselves feel guilty for "what they've done" is the only way to keep themselves on track. Fear of regaining, guilt for 'bad choices" and all sorts of self-flagellation are their motivational tools of choice.

I understand this. We often think that if we don't hold our feet to the fire, we'll just revert to our wildest desires, eating cream puffs by the handful and making a permanent indentation on the couch with our behinds.

Ask any teacher, parent or dog-owner the following question: Is fear a good motivator? Is guilt?

It may work in the short term to get results, but I can promise you this: it won't last. Fear, guilt, and self-recrimination only backfire on us in the long run. No one likes to feel bad and our human tendency is to move away from the things that make us feel bad.

You will not go buck wild and eat 6,000 calories in one day when you start choosing thoughts that make you feel good. On the contrary, you will find it easier to make healthy choices the moment you start making healthy thought choices. What this really comes down to is trusting yourself, and if that's an area you feel very shaky in, that is in an indication of some past programming that needs attention.

Once you have accepted that you are responsible for your own thoughts, and that changing your thoughts will change what you're feeling, you are ready to make some new thoughts.

Chapter 5: Step Three: Replacing Your Thoughts

The creation of new, intentional thinking first requires accepting that we are in control of our thoughts. While at first blush, this may sound obvious and easy; it is often a road block for many people. We sometimes feel like thoughts just "pop into" our heads. These are the automatic thoughts I referred to earlier (like the toe stub), and it's absolutely critical to realize that we have control over changing those thoughts.

Imagine that your thoughts are like a cable package with a number of different channels you can select. As automatic thoughts come in, you can monitor how they make you feel. If you recognize low, negative emotions, you then have a choice to change the channel. Let me give you an example...

Don't think about a giraffe.

What did you think of? I'd be willing to put down some money on the fact that as soon as you read that line, an image of a tall, lumbering giraffe popped into your head before you had time to do anything about it. There's a great example of how powerful our automatic thoughts are. But, if thinking of giraffes caused you pain, guilt, and frustration, the moment you identified those negative feelings you could consciously choose to "change the channel," so to speak, and replace the picture of the giraffe in your head with a thought that created more positive emotions. Like kangaroos, perhaps.

Conscious replacement is just one way to create new intentional thoughts. When a thought pops into your head that creates negative emotions, acknowledge that thought and then choose to replace it with a thought that creates positive emotions. Think of changing your thoughts like changing a channel on a television. You wouldn't tolerate a show you didn't like for very long, so don't tolerate a thought that makes you unhappy or uncomfortable. Often times, an opposite statement is a very simple but direct way to replace your thoughts.

"I feel so fat" is a common automatic thought. This thought might pop into your head as you shop for new clothes, as you walk by a mirror, sit on the beach, go the gym, sit in an uncomfortable chair, look at a picture of yourself, or stand next to a Kate Moss look-a-like in line at the grocery store. Automatic thought, instant negative emotions.

What type of thought might replace "I feel fat" and create more positive emotions? Opposite statements are a good place to start. "I feel healthy" is one example. "I feel thin," "I feel wonderful," and "I feel strong" are some others. Any thought that begins to create a feeling of positive, uplifting, motivating emotions is a good place to start.

But what if the thought "I feel thin" feels like a blatant, bald-faced lie to yourself? This is important. Some new thoughts may create a feeling of doubt. Is doubt a positive or negative emotion? Doubt, or disbelief, in your statement will create more negative emotions and ultimately leaves you with a statement that is too weak to replace your old, powerful thought. Tweaking your new statement to eliminate doubt is an important step in creating new thoughts. Some phrases you can use for minimizing doubt are: "in the process of," "learning to," "on my way to," and any other phrase that describes development or progress. So for example, if "I feel healthy" creates doubt, try "I'm on my way to feeling healthier and healthier."

"I feel thin" becomes "I'm in the process of feeling thinner."

"I love my body" becomes "I am learning to love my body."

"I can do this" becomes "I am on my way to doing this."

The message is the same, but the description of progress instead of an arrival point often allows people the breathing room they need to believe their new thoughts. This is different than creating statements about the future, such as "I will feel healthier" or "I will be thin." A key to the message is the use of present tense. It is easy to fall into the trap of creating new thoughts that talk about what we *will* do or be, tomorrow, next week, next year. When creating new thoughts, we're often tempted to say things like "I will do better tomorrow" or "I will eventually lose this weight!"

Think about the implications of those sentences. For starters, "I will do better tomorrow" implies that you're not doing very well today. What kind of emotion does that generate? "I will eventually lose this weight" implies that at the present moment, you're *not* losing this weight. This is easy to remedy simply by using the process phrases to make the statement describe the present tense. Using future tense can not only make implicit suggestions about what you're doing (or not doing) in the present, but it can also delay the powerful positive emotions you deserve to feel right now!

Conscious replacement is an essential practice for minimizing and erasing old negative thoughts, by replacing these thoughts with new ones that serve you better. Along with replacement, we can also create new thoughts simply by imagining what we would want to be true and scripting dialogue to begin experiencing the emotions that being that way would create. In other words, we don't have to only react to old thoughts, we can create new thoughts just based on what we would like to be true about who we are, what we do and how we feel. I call this *intentional thinking*.

You can approach this by thinking about what you would *like* to be true. For instance, would you like to feel like you had a healthy relationship with food? That you were in control of your choices? Loved your body? Loved to exercise? Begin by visualizing your ideal healthy self, in as many specific ways as possible. How would you feel, how would look, and what would you do if you were the healthiest self you could imagine? Then, using the same process as we did with the conscious replacement, you can script new thoughts around these ideals that feel believable.

If you wanted to have a healthy relationship with food, what might that entail? You could begin to create thoughts like "I choose foods that give me energy." "I crave whole, delicious foods." "I love the taste of fresh fruits and vegetables." Again, if any of these statements create doubt, add in the phrases that indicate that you're in the process of this becoming true. As an example, you might find "I am learning to love the taste of fresh fruits and vegetables" to feel more truthful than the previous statement about produce.

Make sure to make your new thoughts be first person. A sentence like "Vegetables taste good to me" may give you the idea that you want, but the powerful subject of that sentence is the vegetables, not you! Since we're not really too concerned with the emotional well-being of our carrots and spinach, keep yourself as the key focus of each sentence. This journey is about you – your likes, your feelings, and your choices. Not only is it okay to be selfish in your inner monologue, it's necessary!

You also want to shift your thoughts away from describing things you're trying to avoid. For instance, people often come up with thoughts like "I don't eat fried food" or "I won't use chocolate to relieve my stress." Remember my giraffe example? My actual command was "*Don't* think about a giraffe." All your brain had to hear was "giraffe" to create a picture. The other words I used were pretty much meaningless. So when you use "don't eat French fries" as a new thought, what do you think your brain hears? That's right.... FRENCH FRIES! Keep your thoughts focused on what you *will* do, be or feel, rather than giving attention to the very things you're trying to minimize or avoid. It's quite easy to do this. If you come up with a sentence with "don't" "not" or "won't" in it, just ask yourself "So, what will I do?" or "what do I want?" Someone who

52

starts off saying "I won't use chocolate to relieve my stress" can ask the question "So what will I do to relieve my stress?" Their answer might be "I'll use deep breathing to relieve my stress." Or "I'll journal when I'm stressed." (Even better? Get the word "stress" out of the sentence completely, as that's another powerful word you probably don't want to give your attention!)

A powerful intentional thought can be one that has to do with loving your body. This can be a very challenging exercise for many people. Often times, when I'm working with a client I will have them tell me a few things they love about their body. This has turned out to be a very hard activity for people. The only thing one of my clients could come up with the first time we did this exercise was that she had nice ears! (That took her about 5 minutes to come up with and she was nearly in tears by the time she said it.) This can be a really critical piece of programming for people trying to lose weight. You may need to start by modifying the thought, with the process phrases, or by identifying parts of your body that you love, such as your strong arms, or your clear skin, or your healthy heart... or even your nice ears! Begin practicing this new thought, and pay attention to the emotional response you have to this thought.

Another type of intentional thinking we can do has to do with our life circumstances or situations that create stress or discomfort. These are high risk situations for making unhealthy choices with food, exercise, sleep or how we respond to stress.

One of my clients, Nikki, is a stay at home mom of 3 small children under the age of 4. She's told me that among the many challenges of eating healthy and exercising with three little ones at home, the worst time of day for her is late afternoon, after naptimes are over and before her husband comes home. It is during this time of day, while the chaos swirls around her, that she often finds herself seeking respite in a handful of crackers, pretzels or other snack foods. Keeping those foods in the house is important for her, because she wants to be a role model for her children on moderation and not have "off limit" foods that become even more tempting when they are around, but she finds resisting these foods late afternoon is a tremendous struggle for her.

Moving backwards through the TFA Chain, I asked Nikki to back up from the action (snacking) and identify how she's feeling during this mid afternoon time. You can probably imagine some of the things Nikki is feeling around this time – stressed, overwhelmed, exhausted, and frazzled. It's no wonder she's turning to food in that moment to buffer her feelings of stress and frustration!

I asked Nikki to imagine how she would like to be feeling in that moment. After pondering it for a minute, she said she'd like to feel calm, in control, and peaceful. These feelings, she believed, would prevent her from snacking and as an added bonus, would result in a different interaction between Nikki and her husband when he returned from work. Changing her thoughts in this moment would have a long lasting effect on both her health AND her relationship! I asked Nikki what she would have to be thinking in order to feel peaceful, in control and calm in the middle of the mid-afternoon chaos.

Nikki had a really hard time coming up with any intentional thought that she thought would be effective here, so I asked her to see herself from another person's objective view. Temporarily removing yourself from the scene is often a way to clear any resistance to coming up with a new thought. I asked Nikki what she thought someone looking at her world from the outside in might think about her. After some thought, she conceded that a stranger looking in might think Nikki was doing the best she could with a challenging situation, that she was pretty amazing for holding it all together, and she was maybe even a stronger, more competent mother and woman than she realized. I asked her to tell me about the other things she did during the day, the challenges she faced, and what types of things her friends and family members said to her to help her create this picture. From this 3rd person perspective, Nikki was able to derive her first new intentional thought "I'm doing the best I can."

I asked her to walk with me through the TFA Chain with this new thought to try it out. When we got to the "feelings" part, I asked her how that new thought felt. She realized here that the effect wasn't *quite* as powerful as she would need to move her past the much more ingrained old programming. "I'm doing the best I can" felt good, but didn't stop her in her tracks and create a calm and content mind.

Often times it can help to give the new intentional thought a test run, to determine whether or not it's going to be believable and powerful enough to replace the old programming. Remember, you've been practicing this old programming for many years. Creating a powerful thought is essential to diminish the hold that this old programming has on your subconscious.

Nikki and I went back to the thoughts we came up with from her friends and family. As we talked it through, she realized that many of her friends often said things to her like, "Nikki, you are amazing! I don't know how you do it all, but you really do a great job raising your family." Although she had been hearing this from her friends and family, she hadn't really bought into this message for herself because she was so caught up in the day to day stress that raising her three little kids generated.

Nikki decided to start practicing telling herself "I am an amazing mom" – all day long, not just waiting until things got stressful at the end of the day. Eventually, she altered the statement to "I am an amazing woman" and it became her mantra. Of course it did not eliminate the stress of raising her kids, but repeating her mantra all day long helped Nikki remind herself that she *was* doing the best she could with a challenging situation AND created a cue sentence for her to help her recognize when she was turning to food as a response to stress. Nikki reported back to me that after 3 months of using her new intentional thought, she felt more powerful and calm in the middle of the daily "crisis" that she faced. She also reported that while she had not completely eliminated her afternoon snacking, she felt more in control of her choices than she ever had before. The days when she did snack on something mid-afternoon, she often made a healthier choice than she had just 3 months earlier. Her success here inspired her to begin identifying other circumstances that made her feel frustrated and stressed out, and creating new intentional thoughts for each one of those circumstances.

Each one of us has specific sets of circumstances, places or people who can trigger that stress response in us. Whether it is frustration, worry, irritation, anxiety, loneliness, guilt or any other negative emotion, we often react to these circumstances with a set of preprogrammed thoughts that are specific to each situation. Identifying those situations and creating new intentional thoughts for them not only begins to change your everyday programming, but this is also a key component of the second part of Inside Out Weight Management, which is overcoming emotional eating.

Summary: Part I

Before we move on to this second part, let's do a quick recap on programming.

Every action comes from a feeling which comes from a thought. In order to create change in our actions, we need to move backward through the chain and identify the thought that's creating the action. We have a couple of options once we've identified that thought.

We can use *conscious replacement*, by identifying a new, opposite thought to counter the programming that's already there. We can also use *intentional thinking* to create brand-new thoughts based on the ideal self you can envision.

We can use both of these methods in the context of specific circumstances that create negative emotions.

Our new thoughts should be first-person, present-tense and believable. If a thought creates doubt, use an expression that describes progress such as "learning to", "on my way" or "in the process of."

Take your new thought for a test run a few times in order to determine what type of emotion it generates, and if that emotional response will be strong enough to support the action you want to take. Tweak your thought until it is not only believable, but also powerful.

Practice the new thought over and over again. Eventually that thought will begin to permeate your subconscious, until it begins to replace your automatic thoughts. Remember that your automatic thoughts took years to take root, and the change probably won't happen overnight. Stay patient and consistent in your new thought; you can even use reminders such as note cards in visible places or saved in the notes section of your phone, if it helps.

As your new thoughts begin to become a part of your subconscious, you'll notice that actions you've wanted to take start to become easier. This is not because your willpower has changed, it is because you *feel* different. New thoughts create new feelings which support new actions.

If you get stuck, or feel like you're backsliding, pay attention to your thoughts. Chances are they will have reverted to your old, automatic thoughts. Make it your intention to return to your new thoughts, whenever you notice this has happened. With time, this will become much easier to do.

Part II: The 4 Step Process of Overcoming Emotional Eating

Chapter 6: What is Emotional Eating?

On my 20th birthday, I carried boxes full of my stuff into an empty apartment in Durham, NC. I had moved there to do an internship at Duke University, but I didn't know a soul in Durham. My boyfriend and I had just broken up and the rest of my friends were scattered across the East Coast working at internships or taking summer courses.

I was subletting an apartment from a friend of the family and one day, while looking for a flashlight in her storage room, I discovered she had a hidden stash of cookies, crackers and candy.

She hadn't told me that these foods were off-limits, but I innately knew that since they weren't in her cupboards there wasn't exactly an open invitation for me to dig in. When I first discovered the food, I really didn't think too much about it. I had already been to the grocery store, had my foods set up in the fridge and cupboard and really, who was I to be digging into someone's box of Cheez-its?

One night after work, I was sitting in the apartment alone, restless and bored. My only connection to the outside world was my cell phone and Instant Messenger and I had watched every *Friends* and *Seinfeld* rerun possible. As I was watching TV, I found myself headed to her storage closet, like a tractor beam pulling me in, and I grabbed just a handful of Cheez-it. One handful led to another, and soon enough over the course of various nights, I ended up eating her Teddy Grahams, her Wheat Thins and her Oreos. Her STALE Oreos.

Of course, I felt guilty about eating her food and on various grocery store trips I would replenish what I had consumed.

And then I would finish off the replacement.

This behavior felt totally compulsive to me, and I was disgusted and frustrated with myself. I was working at an internship in Employee Health, and was leading a Run/Walk 5k Training program. I was also training for a triathlon, and I knew that my evening snack habits were sabotaging both my healthy weight efforts and my training. I was frustrated and disappointed with myself but I didn't know what to do about it.

I started researching binge eating, but it just didn't seem to fit. I'd stop after 5-6 handfuls of Cheez-its. I wouldn't go on to eat bowls of ice cream, loaves of bread or entire bags of chips. And I didn't have any purging behaviors. I knew I was practicing unhealthy eating habits, but I couldn't seem to find anything in books or online that described what I was experiencing. Not as extreme as binge eating, but a far cry from demonstrating any self control.

I thought I was alone in this struggle until I became a weight loss coach and I spoke to many other people who were going through similar experiences. This is the place where many trying to lose weight find themselves: in the no man's land between healthy eating and binge eating.

My client Jenny has been at the same job for nearly 2 decades and after years of toiling under some stressful but challenging conditions at work, she had landed herself a fairly cushy, low stress management position. Jenny called me because she wanted to become a little bit healthier as she approached her 40th birthday. She's already very active, exercises nearly every day, and makes it a point to eat whole, organic food. But despite nearly every effort she could think of, Jenny found herself succumbing to a bowl of M&Ms on her secretary's desk nearly every day at 10 am. Jenny is a great example of someone caught in the vicious cycle of emotional eating, and I'll tell you how I coached her through breaking the mid-morning chocolate habit.

Emotional eating can impact anyone and the variety of clients I had struggling with this issue illustrates that. Another client of mine, Susie, is retired and divorced, with her 4 grown children living nearby. Her days are busy, full of helping out with her 10 grandchildren, keeping up with her 1-acre garden and volunteering for Meals on Wheels. When Susie first came to me, she wanted to lose 30 pounds. Working together using a calorie budget and a food log (my usual approach to weight loss), Susie lost 27 pounds in a little over 7 months. However, as we neared her goal of 30 lbs, Susie found herself backsliding. She'd go all day long making healthy food choices and exercising and felt great. But nearly every night, she'd describe having overpowering snack cravings. She tried to control these cravings by removing the candy, chips, and ice cream from her house but found that she still overate with fruit, almonds, cheese or popcorn.

These two examples, along with my personal example, provide a few illustrations of what emotional eating might look like. Emotional eating feels very compulsive and automatic to the person experiencing it. Some people describe it as a separation of mind and body: the mind is telling you not to eat, but the hands seem to keep on lifting the fork or spoon to the mouth. This type of eating often occurs standing up, when the person is alone, and frequently at night. It is rarely an instance of being legitimately hungry.

For most people, emotional eating creates feelings of guilt, frustration, irritation and helplessness. People describe it as self-sabotage, and they often feel powerless to stop the behavior. A few of my clients have told me they *enjoy* the behavior, but they recognize it's preventing them from achieving their healthy lifestyle goals.

To begin with, let's define emotional eating. Emotional eating is a disconnection. It is the act of removing yourself from a situation that creates discomfort but has no easy remedy. Let's say you are sitting in your living room watching TV and you realize you're cold. What would you do? You might get up and turn on the heat, or put on a sweater, or get a blanket. So although you are experiencing an uncomfortable situation, it is easily remedied.

Now, as a contrast, I'll walk you through a similar scenario of a situation that creates discomfort, but doesn't have an easy remedy. It's the end of a long day. Throughout your busy day, you've dealt with a lot of different challenges and stresses – the demands of your job, some financial interactions, dealing with your children or spouse, and maybe some worries about your health. None of these are top of mind right now, the only thing you're conscious of paying attention to is selecting your favorite show from the DVR. You sit down to relax in front of the show, and as you do, some of these stressors of the day begin to float into your subconscious mind. Maybe it's the nagging of an unpaid bill. Thinking about what's still on your desk at work waiting for you tomorrow. Wondering about what you're going to do about your aging parents. Whatever that thought might be, it creates a feeling of worry, stress or tension. Or maybe there is loneliness. Or boredom. Any of these emotions create a feeling of discomfort, but none of them are as easily remedied as getting up and putting on a sweater or cranking up the heat. Imagine if you sat there and dwelled upon these emotions for the rest of the evening. Whether it was worry, fear, frustration, loneliness or even boredom – to sit there and dwell upon these feelings would render you nearly non-functional.

By disconnecting, your subconscious mind is actually protecting you. In the exact moment that you start thinking about what type of ice cream might be in your freezer or whether or not there are any Pringles left in your pantry, you are essentially removing yourself from those emotions or from that uncomfortable situation that has no easy remedy. As soon as you are in action – scooping out the ice cream or opening the bag of chips – you experience the rewarding, calming effect of instant gratification coupled with removal from a negative experience. So while our conscious mind may be saying "Are you sure you want to be doing this?" our subconscious mind pushes on full steam ahead.

This is a process that is usually learned early on, most likely in childhood. Our very first experience with food is typically a positive one, associated with the comfort of being held by our mothers. Then as we grow into small children, food is often used as a reward: for being quiet, for behaving well, for good grades, even for eating other less appealing foods! Practice the behavior of food being a reward for many years, and it's no wonder that so many people experience a strong, positive rush of emotions when they remove themselves from an uncomfortable situation with food.

The types of food we crave when we're emotionally eating hold a key to understanding this behavior as well. I know very few people who crave baby carrots or lush, green Granny Smith apples when they're eating as a response to their emotions. For most people, "comfort foods" fall into three main categories: sweet foods, salty & crunchy foods, or creamy, heavy foods. This makes sense, from an evolutionary perspective. When food was not nearly as plentiful as it is today, obtaining and storing calories was a means of survival. Both high sugar and high fat foods would have been calorically dense, so it stands to reason that we would be predisposed to want to eat high volumes of these foods when we come across them. Salt, a mineral essential for survival, was also not as readily available as it is today and would have been equally as important for consumption. Not only are we reinforced to eat by our emotional response, but we are physiologically primed for it as well.

In my experience, emotional eating has been the most common barrier that holds someone back from achieving his or her weight loss goals. A very small percentage of people who want to lose weight simply need to know how many calories their body needs and how many calories are in the foods they consume, and they are off and losing weight almost effortlessly. The overwhelming majority of those with whom I worked were experiencing some level of emotional eating that was holding them back from where they wanted to be.

Most other weight loss programs I've tried or reviewed fall short when it comes to dealing with emotional eating. The typical response to emotional eating is to find a new reaction to the uncomfortable situation. For instance, if someone said that she ate when she was stressed, a common solution would be to offer advice such as going for a walk, calling a friend, or listening to calming music. While all of these are good strategies for mediating stress relief, they do not, in my experience, seem to work as a long-term solution. If the situation that is generating stress is chronic or intense enough, we will ultimately go back to the more ingrained, practiced method of stress relief: disconnecting with food.

Food is an extremely reliable and easy mechanism for disconnection. It is available just about everywhere we go: our homes, our offices, our cars, our shopping centers, airports, movie theatres, sporting events and practically every social event we attend. There is even food available in my gym if I want it! In fact, the only place I can think of where I spend any time that doesn't have food available is the dog park. We would have an extremely difficult time removing food from the places we spend our time, and removing food from our social interactions with others. Besides the fact that food is present nearly everywhere we go, there's one other small barrier to trying to remove food from our lives: *we need it to survive.* Food is relatively inexpensive, extremely convenient and part of our social fabric. Simply put, we must relearn a healthier relationship with food and learn to exist in a world where the object of our disconnection is going to be present nearly all the time.

Emotional eating is best approached from the inside out. Rather than trying to replace eating with another action, my approach works to identify, change and minimize the triggers that cause disconnection in the first place. This approach is a four-step process that is easy to follow and, when used consistently, is extremely effective. But best of all, it is freedom from the cravings that have haunted nearly every person who has attempted to gain control over his or her eating.

Rather than trying to tackle emotional eating with an action, I lead my clients through a process that approaches emotional eating from the inside out. We work on first identifying the thought that generates the feeling that triggers the action (eating.) Changing this pathway is an easy to follow and simple to use four step process. It is quite similar to the Inside Out Weight Management process, and they can easily be used at the same time.

Chapter 7: Step One: Awareness

The first step is awareness.

Recognizing the moments in which you're experiencing an episode of emotional eating is critical to creating change. Typically, people feel very limited control over the type of food that they are choosing, or the portion sizes that they have. They may say "I am just going to have a half a cup of ice cream" and then find themselves going back for another, and another...and another... Or, one handful of crackers becomes three or four handfuls. Eight almonds become eighty almonds. They have limited control over how much they have or what type of food they have, as you saw in my example of my raiding the storage closet at my apartment and diving into stale Oreos!

The food or the portion size itself is not the defining characteristics of an episode of emotional eating. Plenty of people can eat large bowls of ice cream, or have four handfuls of crackers and it may be a conscious decision. The key distinction to recognizing an episode of emotional eating is the feeling of a lack of control over the situation and the accompanying emotions of guilt, disappointment or frustration that occur either while you're eating or immediately afterwards.

The first step in our four step process of overcoming emotional eating is awareness. Awareness is recognizing when emotional eating is happening. The only action you have to take to complete the first step is to catch yourself in the moment. If you're alone, or with friends or family who won't judge you, even say out loud to yourself something like "I'm emotionally eating RIGHT NOW!" Like I said, this is best reserved for moments alone or with open-minded companions. Shouting that sentence when you're digging into the free sugar cookie display at the grocery store may earn you some strange looks from passers-by.

Awareness is key. Emotional eating is typically a subconscious behavior, and changing it requires lifting it from the subconscious to the conscious. Awareness itself can play an important role in changing our eating behaviors, as our food choices are often made mindlessly and as a result of purely ingrained habitual behavior.

To be clear, there are occasions when one can overeat and it may *not* be emotional eating. For instance, there are a number of different "cues" that can trigger eating that may or may not have anything to do with our emotional state. One such type of cues is called "visual cues." Have you ever been driving down the highway on a long road trip and see a billboard with a nice, juicy hamburger and suddenly found yourself looking for the nearest exit? This is an example of a visual cue. The *sight* of food, even a picture of food, can trigger the urge to eat. This can happen with TV commercials, it can happen when your coworker brings brownies into the office and you happen to stumble upon them in the break room, and it can happen when you walk by a bustling bakery on your way to work. These situations are different from emotional eating, although it's equally as important to be aware of them when they happen too! Besides sight, other senses can trigger cues to eat. The buttery smell of popcorn when you walk into the movie theater triggers a strong craving for anyone – even if you've just had dinner!

There are other types of cues called "conditioned responses." Think of Pavlov and his dogs, who were conditioned to respond to the sound of a bell with a salivating response, after numerous exposures of the bell paired with food. We are conditioned like Pavlov's dog to pair many different experiences with food as well. For instance, most people associate certain foods with attending a baseball game or walking into a movie theater. Sometimes these experiences are tied in with emotions, but this is not always the case. Holiday foods are often a conditioned response, but for many people, there's an emotional tie to them as well.

The key to recognizing emotional eating is the feeling of a lack of control over your choices, and the feelings of guilt, disappointment or frustration that occur either while you're eating or immediately afterwards. If you're having trouble determining whether or not you are experiencing emotional eating, I've included a list of questions in the appendix that you can use to help you explore your food habits and choices.

Chapter 8: Step Two: Asking the Question

This second step in the four step process of combating emotional eating is called "asking the question." The question that you ask yourself once you recognize that you are experiencing emotional eating is *"what am I disconnecting from?"* Asking this question will help you identify what emotion or uncomfortable situation you are using food to distract or pacify yourself.

Asking the question also serves to create a pause, during which you move yourself from subconscious actions to conscious awareness. By creating awareness, you can diminish behaviors of impulse and act with more logical thought. Most of the time, these behaviors are so automatic you almost don't realize you are doing them!

At first, the question simply needs to be asked, in that moment where emotional eating is occurring. It can be asked before you're eating, while you're eating, or while you're standing there licking your finger to get the last pieces of salt from the now-empty bag of potato chips. It doesn't matter *when* you ask (for now), as long as you get in the habit of asking the question.

If you're alone, ask the question out loud. Hearing your voice out loud asking the question will create an even greater effect of moving to conscious thought. If you are with understanding, supportive people (spouses, family or friends), let them know what you're going to be doing and why. As a final option, you can simply ask the question in your head. There's no right or wrong way to do this; this step is simply about *doing*. Ask the question and create awareness.

For many people, this step alone can begin to change habits. It's not usually powerful enough to create long-term effects, but the simple act of bringing a level of consciousness to a formerly mindless task does begin to alter behavior. While it's important to keep going through the process, don't be surprised if you start to notice changes at this step.

For one of my clients, Kelli, this step alone was a turning point for her. Kelli is a stay at home mom to 4 teens and felt like her house full of teenage-friendly snacks and crazy schedule was keeping her from making any headway with her weight loss goals. Kelli was grazing all day long at home, and we started off by trying to create a more structured eating schedule to make sure we addressed her hunger levels. When this didn't curb her snacking, we started exploring the emotional eating aspect of Kelli's snacking. When we got to this step, Kelli decided she was going to ask herself "Why do I want to eat that?" and give herself 10 minutes to pause before she committed to snacking. She decided if the 10 minutes passed and she still wanted it, she would go ahead and eat it. Kelli was so surprised to report 2 weeks later, that most of the time she would get caught up in doing something else while waiting for her 10-minutes to pass and would forget about the snack. When she didn't, she would try to answer the question and identify what was going on before going ahead and having the snack. Eventually, we were able to identify that Kelli was often bored and lonely at home during the day and was snacking as a way to disconnect from these feelings. It took awhile for Kelli to realize this because her "to do list" was so long she couldn't have imagined that boredom was the root of her behavior. However, even before she was able to identify what exactly was prompting her to eat, just asking the question and giving herself time to pause before having something to eat was enough to begin the process of creating some behavior change. This in turn excited and motivated Kelli enough to keep working through the next steps.

Chapter 9: Step Three: Analyze the Answers

The third step in the four step process to combating emotional eating is "analyze the answers." Once you have practiced and created the habit of asking yourself the question "What am I disconnecting from?" you will begin to answer the question. In doing so, you will be gathering information that will be critical to releasing you from the cycle of emotional eating. As you answer the question, gather the information in one place: on an index card in your wallet, a post-it note on your desk, a text message or email you send to yourself, or a small notebook you carry with you. Even if you think you will remember what you're coming up with, writing it down is strongly encouraged to transition into the next step.

As you collect the answers, you can begin to analyze them for trends. Themes may begin to appear in your answers, whether it is certain places, people, times of day or situations that are triggers for your moments of disconnection. I find that most people can narrow down their list to two or three main "triggers" of disconnection.

My client Jenny, who craved M&Ms every morning at 10 am, discovered she was bored at work. On a typical day, she arrived at work around 8 am, would go through her to do list, answer all her emails and get all her menial work out of the way first. Around 10 am, she would decide what project she was going to work on that day. In that moment, as she pondered how she would spend her workday, Jenny was subconsciously realizing that she was truly unhappy in her job. As I mentioned earlier, Jenny had worked under some very stressful conditions but had recently been moved into a more comfortable, relaxing management position. It really wasn't in her conscious thoughts that she would want to leave or change the position she had worked so hard to earn, so dwelling on her boredom created some very real discomfort for Jenny. She recognized, by asking the question, that she was using the candy to disconnect from the discomfort of not being very happy in her job. Exploring this topic was very hard for Jenny. She was afraid to admit to herself that she wasn't happy in the job, because she wasn't sure what that meant. Should she be looking for another one? Did she want to go back to the other position she had, even though it was so stressful? She had thought, as she toiled away at her old position, that this comfortable management position was the reward that was waiting for her. Acknowledging that she was unhappy now went against the beliefs she had held for most of her job career. Jenny wasn't ready to think or talk about this. So every time the thoughts threatened to break into the conscious realm, to the candy jar she went. As she went to the candy jar, the thought of "mmm, chocolate!" quickly replaced "What am I doing here?"

This step was even more challenging for Susie. Susie's emotional eating occurred at night, after dinner. As she went through the process, she began to realize that she was disconnecting from the loneliness that settled in after a long day. While she was busy tending to her grandchildren, her garden, her church members or her children, she didn't have time to focus on herself and how lonely she felt. Susie told me that she and her husband used to sit on their front porch at the end of every day and talk about what was going on in their lives. It didn't take long for her to connect the dots and realize that her snacking at night was a disconnection from the loneliness she felt from missing this ritual. Dealing with this loneliness felt so overwhelming to Susie that she told me at one point, "I think I'd rather just keep eating than face the loneliness."

Loneliness and boredom were the culprits in my emotional eating as well. Although I had plenty of friends available by cell phone and Instant Messenger, I hadn't yet met anyone in Durham to spend time with after work. I wasn't really conscious of being lonely because I was still using Instant Messenger to be in constant contact with friends, but, obviously, that wasn't sufficient, and I was disconnecting from the uncomfortable feeling of loneliness with my late night snacking.

In the third step, as you analyze the answers, you begin to notice if there were certain people, places or situations that frequently occurred during or before the moment when you're disconnecting. For some people, it might be interactions with certain people – maybe a coworker or family member – that often precede patterns of emotional eating. It could also be that you notice your patterns of emotional eating tend to happen most when you're in certain places, such as at work, parties or other social gatherings or visiting someone else's home. Emotional eating can also be triggered by certain situations such as stressful conversations, a daily task or a specific activity. Recognizing those patterns can help you determine what situations are triggering uncomfortable emotional states that you are using food to disconnect from. This step is critical before moving on to the final step.

Before moving on to the final step, I'll recap the first three steps one more time. The first step in the process of combating emotional eating is awareness. Awareness is recognizing when you're experiencing emotional eating, by paying attention to how you feel while you're eating or shortly after. Emotional eating feels compulsive and often times involves eating large portions, eating by yourself, and eating at times when you aren't physically hungry. There are times when you may meet these criteria, but eating does not feel compulsive. When you know that you have consciously chosen to eat this way, then that is not an example of emotional eating.

The second step is asking the question "what am I disconnecting from?" This question serves to create a pause that moves you from subconscious to conscious behavior. Emotional eating is often a subconscious behavior, and asking a question requires you to become more attentive to the moment and raises you into your conscious-level thinking. Behavior change may start here, but it is still critical to keep moving forward through all the steps.

The third step is to analyze the answer to the question, write it down and look for repetitious themes such as people, places or situations that trigger emotional eating.

Chapter 10: Step Four: Adjust Your Thinking

The fourth and final step of overcoming emotional eating is called "Adjust your Thinking." Adjusting your thinking relies on the TFA process that we discussed in Part One. As discussed earlier, TFA stands for "Thoughts, Feelings and Actions." Thoughts create feelings, feelings create actions. When most people try to lose weight they focus solely on changing their actions, or behaviors, and they are usually unsuccessful in maintaining those behavior changes for a long time.

Because actions stem from feelings and feelings stem from thoughts, until an individual changes their thoughts, they will continue to fight against themselves and exhaust their willpower. Like we did with reprogramming, we'll focus on changing thoughts to change the emotions that are triggering the cravings and decision to eat. Eventually, this will reduce or eliminate using food as an emotional response. Let's take Jenny as an example, whose main thought in her trigger was "I'm bored and I don't really enjoy my job."

Once Jenny had identified her thoughts (through step 3, "Analyze your Answers"), we moved on to explore what feelings this thought was creating. For Jenny, thinking about how she wasn't very happy with her job made her feel frustrated, bored and most importantly, fearful. The fear existed because Jenny didn't know what else she would do if she didn't do *this* job, a position she had worked hard to get to and a position that came with a lot of perks. Boredom, frustration and fear – all uncomfortable emotions without easy remedies. As soon as these thoughts threatened to surface in her conscious mind, her brain would switch over to thoughts of "Chocolate! Chocolate! Must find chocolate!"

This is an appropriate time to point out that disconnection is, in actuality, a protective mechanism. The reason it is such a stubborn behavior to change is that, on some level, disconnection is actually helping you. By focusing on the thoughts of chocolate, Jenny removes herself from those uncomfortable emotions. Over time, we subconsciously learn that focusing on food can protect us from experiencing negative emotions. However, this effect is temporary and does nothing to actually address the situation that is creating the discomfort in the first place. Jenny frequently tried to address this behavior by bringing fruit to substitute, or getting up to take a walk, or even just mentally beating herself up, but her attention was focused on changing the action without identifying what was *driving* the action.

Once we've identified the thought and feelings driving the action, we can now work backwards through the chain to try and change the situation. I asked Jenny what action she would like to take, and she said "well, I would like to work through the morning until 10 o'clock when I have a healthy snack of my own choosing."

I asked her what emotional state she would have to be in order to make a healthy choice and she identified that she'd have to be feeling satisfied, content and engaged.

From there, we move one step backwards again and I asked her what thought would have to be present in her mind in order to feel satisfied, content and engaged. This is the time of day that Jenny was focused on more menial tasks, like responding to emails and creating her "to do list" for the day. It was difficult for her to imagine how she might feel accomplished or engaged at this point in the day, without a project to work on.

Part of changing this situation for Jenny involved identifying a project that would make her feel engaged and satisfied with her job. Although Jenny's prior role at work was more stressful, she felt challenged and excited by the projects she worked on. Jenny and I brainstormed what were the characteristics of her old job she had enjoyed, and how she could recreate those characteristics in her new role. She realized that one of the things she had loved most about her old role was interacting with people and identifying ways to improve their working conditions. In her new role in a management position, she didn't have as much interaction on a day to day basis with the people she was in charge of, but she did create training materials and educational information for them. Thinking about this project in the framework of helping others and making their jobs easier helped Jenny tap into the feelings of satisfaction and enjoyment that she was missing in her new role.

At 10 am, as Jenny looked to starting her project, she'd intentionally practice thinking "I am helping the new hires. I am making their lives easier." When we practiced this, Jenny felt optimistic that if she could create that mindset, she would create more positive emotions at work. As is often the case, identifying ways to change your thinking may ultimately end up creating changes in your life too. Sometimes it is effective enough to change your perception of a situation, and in other cases changing your thoughts help you recognize the situation itself needs to be changed. This ended up being true for Jenny. Ultimately her long-term happiness at work required her to change both the day to day flow of her workday as well as taking on different types of projects and redefining what her role was at work. However, all of this *started* with Jenny changing her thoughts.

This type of thinking is called *intentional thinking*. Remember the toe stub? Jenny's automatic thinking is about her boredom, so in order for this step to work she will have to intentionally choose to think this new thought. I like to call this step "fake it til you make it." The new thought may feel a little bit unnatural, forced or even ineffective at first. You'll have to remember that your old, automatic thoughts about a situation have had much longer to be ingrained as truth in your brain than this new thought. But you will begin to believe ANY thought if you choose to think it over and over again. So "fake it til you make it." Practice this new thought with intention until it begins to feel true, and creates the emotions that you want to feel.

Just like in reprogramming, your new thoughts will be most effective if they are in the present tense and first person. Also, if you find they are creating doubt, you can use the modifiers we talked about in Part I such as "in the process of" "learning to" or "beginning to."

Over time as you replace the old thought with the new thought, the new one will begin to permeate the subconscious. As it does, the situations, people or places that may have formerly triggered negative emotions will either cease to be triggers for emotional eating or will greatly diminish in their effect. Not only will you be changing your eating habits, but you may also notice that this helps minimize the stress that these situations cause you in the first place.

Summary: Part II

The process of working through emotional eating is one you may have to return to again and again before it begins to be something you can work through with relative ease and confidence. Before we go on to explore a few more ways to refine the experience of Inside Out Weight Management, I'll go through a summary of the four steps to overcoming emotional eating. This summary can be used as a quick way to refresh yourself whenever you need it.

The first step is simply awareness. Catching yourself in the act of emotional eating and making it something you are consciously aware of doing is the first step to creating change. Acknowledging the behavior while you are in the midst of it happening can accomplish this. There are situations where you may overeat or even feel guilty about overeating that may not be emotional eating so it's important to recognize your own patterns and behaviors. I provided a list of questions in the appendix that could be a useful tool for determining whether or not you are experiencing emotional eating.

The second step is "ask the question." Once you've begun to create awareness around the times you are emotionally eating, you can begin asking yourself "What am I disconnecting from?" You can come up with any phrase you like that sounds good to your ears, but the intention is to ask yourself a question that will serve as a pause before you start eating. It can be helpful during this step to write down your answers, maybe on an index card or in the notes section of your phone.

This will give you some information to refer back to during the third step.

The third step to overcoming emotional eating is "analyze the answers." This is the step where you look for patterns in your behavior, such as what emotions you were experiencing before eating, where you were, what time of day it was or who you were with. Using the information that you gathered in step two, you can begin to figure out your emotional eating triggers. Most people tend to identify a few consistent triggers.

The fourth and final step is "adjust your thinking." It is during this step that we use the TFA process to change the thoughts that are ultimately the real cause of emotional eating. Some of the strategies discussed for adjusting your thinking include the use of phrases like "in the process of" or "starting to" as well as the use of opposite statements. The key to creating powerful new thoughts was to make them believable, as well as to state them in the first-person and present tense.

These four steps are the foundation for working through emotional eating. Using them as well as the Inside Out Weight Management process outlined in Part I are the keys to creating sustainable and meaningful behavior change. They are the basics of behavior change and it may be useful to refer back to them on a regular basis. In the next few chapters, we'll explore a few more ways to expand upon these strategies and make them even more powerful.

Chapter 11: Putting it to Work

Shoot, I need to get an oil change. I wonder when I can go. Maybe Thursday? No, definitely not Thursday, I've got a doctor's appointment Thursday and that meeting is on Friday so I better leave some time to prepare for that. I'm so not prepared for that. I need to email Joe and see where the numbers are for that. I wonder if our tax return is ready yet. I need to pay our water bill I think. Crap, I need to get to the grocery store, too. I don't know what I'm cooking for dinner tonight. Maybe I'll just get pizza. That's not very healthy though, can't eat that. But, blech, I'm so sick of chicken. I need to lose some weight. These pants are way too tight. I hate the way they look. I hate the way I LOOK. I need to go to the gym. My knee hurts. I wonder who's going to get kicked off American Idol tonight. I'm so tired. I shouldn't have stayed up so late watching TV last night.

What? Don't tell me you haven't heard a similar dialogue play in *your* own head before?

Whenever I stop to actually pay attention to the running stream of consciousness in my head, I often find if I'm not monitoring it, it's like having an email inbox with no spam filters. It's a free for all of thoughts, with no limitations on what I actually *want* there.

We just determined that the thoughts we have will create our emotions, which will dictate our actions. Since we're all constantly in the process of thinking, the idea of monitoring each and every one of those thoughts in order to play the "bait and switch" game to stay on track with positive, helpful thoughts can be completely overwhelming.

So how do you use the process of intentional thinking in your busy day-to-day life?

There's a simple way to monitor whether or not your thoughts are on track to support the healthy actions you want to be making and that, as I've mentioned before, is to monitor your feelings. When you find yourself feeling anything negative such as stress, anxiety, boredom, loneliness, or frustration, that is a **clear** signal that your thoughts are headed in the wrong direction.

Once you recognize that you're experiencing negative emotions, you're in a position to do something about it. This is the game I call "The Catch." I call it that because the first step is catching yourself in the moment of having a negative thought... or thoughts. I often notice physical cues that I'm getting into negativity mode – an uneasy, tense feeling in the pit of my stomach, or I'll find my hand has flown up to rub the back of my neck. Or, of course, an overwhelming desire to turn the car immediately into the nearest coffee drive through and get a mocha frappe.

I slam the brakes on my thoughts (and my car) as soon as I catch myself in the experience of negative emotions and immediately ask myself this question: **So, what DO I want?**

It's an easy question to answer, and as soon as I shift from what I **don't want**, what I **lack**, what I **fear**, what I **worry** about to start focusing on what I **hope for**, what I have **plenty** of, what I **celebrate**, what I am **confident** in, the change in my mood is immediate. My focus shifts to gratitude, optimism, excitement and peace of mind. The knot in my stomach releases, the tension disappears from my neck and my car stays on its due course. When you focus on what you want, you start feeling hopeful and then noticing when you're getting what you want. When you focus on what you have plenty of, you wallow in gratitude and the feeling of security. When you start celebrating, you find joy in the every day. Focusing on the positive is hardly a concept anyone can argue against for better living and it doesn't have to be so difficult. Just catch yourself in the act of negative self-talk and then ask: "What do I want?"

I've worked with clients on the process of changing their thoughts and they'll say something like, "I'll have to figure out when I can fit that in my day." What? You're ALWAYS thinking... you can fit this in your day ALL THE TIME. But I know it's not that simple. Sometimes you just don't feel like you have the power to change your thoughts. And sometimes, despite a good effort, our thoughts can feel totally stuck on the negative. It feels like everything is happening *to you* and you're just putting out fires and running from one crisis to the next.

When you're feeling that way, there's a back-up plan for changing your thoughts. It's outrageously simple but incredibly effective. When you are so overcome by negative thoughts that you feel incapable of adjusting them, begin to focus simply on your breathing. Breathe in and out through your nose, and try to breathe as slowly as possible. As you breathe, begin to match the inhalation and expiration with a two-word phrase with one-syllable words, or one word with two syllables.

Here are a few I love: "I Am." "Let Go." "Be Still."

Here are a few my clients have come up with: "Calm Down." "Oh-Kay." "Strong-ger." "All good."

I stumbled upon this strategy when I first started trying to meditate. After years of practice, I can finally meditate on nothing but silence. But when I first started trying, every time I would try to get quiet and just listen to the sound of my breath, I would find that an ocean of thoughts would come crashing down on me almost immediately. After a few minutes of trying to wipe my mind clean, only to have those thoughts come rushing back in, I would give up, totally frustrated. I felt like I had no absolutely no power over my mind.

One book I read on meditation introduced me to the idea of using a mantra while I meditated. Immediately, I found this to be very effective. Using the mantra gave my mind something to focus on, without really focusing on anything. Over time, I found that I could choose messages that were appropriate for the effect I wanted to achieve. I often use them when I'm driving in the car, sitting at work, or right before I fall asleep – the times where I tend to notice my mind wandering the most.

I use "Let Go" when I'm replaying a situation that didn't go the way I wanted to over and over in my head. I use "Be Still" when I'm anxious about something in the future, and I want to feel calmer. But my favorite is "I Am." I use this one in all types of situations and it quickly and effectively calms my mind.

Using the manta paired with breath is a simple way to push the negative thoughts out of your mind. Over time, you'll find that as you do this, you'll begin to make space in your mind where you can create new positive thoughts to take root. I like to think of mantras as a way to sweep the rooms of the mind clean, where they sit ready and waiting for whatever you *choose* to put in them.

Using the process of "The Catch" and the breathing with a mantra are two simple ways to begin to practice gaining control over your thoughts. Recognizing that you, and only you, have control over your mind is the cornerstone to being able to effectively use intentional thinking. If you find that you're struggling with the steps introduced in the earlier parts of this book, this is a great place to start to help you begin to feel a greater sense of control over your own thoughts.

These exercises will stretch you and strengthen you just like any physical exercise would. The more often you practice them, the stronger you will grow in your capability to choose your desired thoughts. The more often you consciously choose positive thoughts, the more likely those types of thoughts are to permeate your subconscious and become rooted in your mind, such that *they* become your new automatic thoughts. Once that happens, you'll be able to maintain your weight loss and overcome your cravings with significantly greater ease than before.

This has been one of the most successful exercises I've introduced to clients. I've been especially excited to see the changes that it has elicited in people who swore they had no self-control over their thoughts or felt like their minds were constantly racing. I've had clients who try this report that they are sleeping better and that they become less reactive in situations that normally triggered stressful or emotional reactions. It's probably one of the simplest exercises I've ever learned myself or shared with others, and yet it is one of the most powerful and effective stress management tools.

Chapter 12: Dealing with Stress

I have found that one of the most common triggers for emotional eating is stress. Stress seems to be an epidemic lately; almost everyone I know talks about how stressed they are. Since so many people are experiencing stress and it has such a huge impact on the food choices we make, it's worth spending some time examining what stress is and how we can address it.

Our body reacts to stress with what is called the "fight or flight response." As a leftover survival mechanism, your body literally prepares itself to fight or run away. Your heart rate goes up, blood pressure is elevated and a cascade of adrenaline is released throughout your body. In layman's terms, it's how you feel when you're "on edge." Back in our caveman days, this type of reaction was very useful because stress might have come about as a result of having to square off with a hungry saber tooth tiger. In other words, our stress then came as a result of acute bouts of stress that threatened our literal survival. We still experience stress like this. For instance, the way you feel when you have to slam on the brakes to nearly avoid a car accident is a good example of the effects of "fight or flight." The nausea in the pit of your stomach and the way your hands shake for a few minutes after the event are the effects of the stress hormones that were just released throughout your body. We still have moments of acute stress and that adrenaline rush can help us react to those moments with greater speed or strength than we would have otherwise. If you're thinking about the typical anecdote of a mom lifting a car off her child, you're on the right track.

Most of our stress these days, however, is more chronic, persistent, long-term stress that doesn't have an easy remedy. Examples might be the daily demands of our job, caring for children or aging parents, worrying over money or relationships, feeling strapped for time, or worrying about our health. While these are all chronic, long-term stressors, our body still reacts in a similar manner as it did in our caveman days.

While acute stress is generally the result of an experience, such as slamming on the brakes of your car, chronic stress is generally the result of *thinking about* experiences. Furthermore, usually when you're thinking, you're often thinking about either the past or the future. We may be dwelling on a situation that didn't go the way we would have liked it to go, or pondering something in the future and worrying over what might happen. *Is it going to get worse? How will I handle it? What should I do? What will they say?*

Rarely do you feel stress when you are focused on the present moment. In fact, being present is what many experts call "being mindful" or "finding flow." If you ever have one of those moments when you're working on something and you're so focused and engaged on it that time seems to just slip right by, then you are in the present moment. You can be present with tasks that require concentration such as writing, working, crafting, cooking, playing a musical instrument or engaging in physical activity. But you can just as easily experience it with repetitious tasks such as washing dishes, swimming laps, waxing your car or hitting a bucket of golf balls at the driving range. When you are engaged and in the present, you are no longer thinking about the past or future sources of your stress.

This is why food is often used as a way of disconnecting from stress. When you are thinking about what to eat, focused on what you are eating, or thinking about what you have *just* eaten, you have effectively ceased to stop thinking about whatever was causing your stress before. However, as we all know, this effect is only temporarily and often is followed by a new source of stress: guilt and frustration that you just overate.

While I've given you an effective means of addressing emotional eating, it can be even more powerful to attend to the stress itself. Less stress means less stress eating! As I said before, the type of stress we experience most often is chronic stress brought about by thinking about past or future experiences. It can be challenging to rein in our thinking.

When my dog and I set out on our morning walk, he is eager to explore and strains forward against the leash even though time and time again, I pull him back beside me. Sometimes I feel like I have to do this every few minutes! At times, I get so frustrated with him, wondering why he can't just stay right beside me. Our minds are just like this, constantly pulling in many directions, getting distracted by all the stimulus around us, and having to be reined back in on a regular basis.

There are a myriad of ways to rein your thoughts in when you recognize that you are dwelling on something that is causing you stress. One of the most effective ways, which I addressed earlier, is to focus on your breathing. When you start focusing on your breathing, and even using the 2-word mantra, you shift your thoughts away from the source of stress. Focusing on the breath immediately brings you back to the present moment and can create a state of calmness. There's even a physical impact: slow, deep breathing helps lower the heart rate and even temporarily lowers blood pressure.

Another way to shift your thoughts from stress-generating thoughts is to start talking to yourself about what you're doing *right now*. For example, if I notice that I'm getting caught up thinking about something stressful, I will start narrating what I'm doing: "I'm driving the car. I'm holding the wheel. I'm sitting in the seat. I'm turning left." It sounds silly but in doing this, you are intentionally redirecting your mind to the present moment and noting your external surroundings.

Sometimes stress itself is a source of stress! This is called "piggyback stress." When you hear someone say, "I know I shouldn't be worried about this" or "I need to stop beating myself up about this" you are hearing piggyback stress. There is the initial stress – the worry or the guilt – and then the associated stress that we have created about having negative feelings in the first place!

While it may feel like the only way to solve an issue that is causing your stress or to prevent a past mistake from reoccurring is to keep thinking about it until you come up with a solution, this is not usually the case. For some people, the idea of shifting their thoughts away from their sources of stress feels like burying their heads in the sand. They worry if that if they don't *worry* about things, the problems will get worse. I am certainly not encouraging you to ignore issues that need resolution. However, in most cases, when we are ruminating on things we are not in a creative or productive frame of mind to create solutions. To many people's surprise, it is often when they *let go* of thinking about their sources of stress that the solutions to these situations come to them. I once asked one of my friends, who rarely seemed to get stressed, how he handled his problems. His answer was: "If I can't come up with a solution in 5 minutes, I know now is not the time to be thinking about it. I let it go and come back to it later."

I think we can all agree that the best decisions are not made when your mind is racing and you're not thinking clearly. Letting go of stress-causing thoughts doesn't mean ignoring issues that need your attention, such as bills to be paid, decisions to be made, or health to be addressed. It simply means acknowledging that at this moment you are not currently in a healthy and productive mind frame to problem solve and choosing to refocus your mind to decrease your stress. This is especially imperative when stress is a trigger for unhealthy behaviors, such as overeating.

Chapter 13: Relapse

The process is not fail proof, and at some point, you will probably hit a roadblock. For almost every one of my clients, and for myself, creating this type of change was a journey made up of some successes and some setbacks. Be prepared for the setbacks, but more importantly, try to understand them.

I used this process pretty successfully myself for almost two years before I had a major relapse. I had had a few smaller setbacks, a bad day here, or an off week there, but it wasn't until right after Christmas 2009 that I experienced a huge setback. Ironically, I was in the middle of writing this book and considered whether or not everything I had learned for myself, believed in and taught to others had just been a lie.

Shortly after Christmas, I started feeling like a dark storm cloud was over my head all the time. I was frustrated with a particular situation that was going on in my professional life, but the bad mood I was in was really disproportionate to my work situation. My fuse was short, and I kept finding more and more things to add to my list of reasons to be stressed out. I felt like a magnet for stress! I knew I was creating my stressful reactions by dwelling on negative thoughts, but I felt like I was stuck in a vicious cycle that I couldn't break. I kept telling myself I had to get out of this funk, and I knew I needed to practice all the techniques I had developed in order to do so.

I kept trying to change my thoughts, but I found the effect would only last a day or two before I would catch myself returning back to my old, negative thoughts and obsessing over the things that were upsetting me. I tried to go to my back up plan: breathing. It had worked for me many times in the past, and I expected it to work again. I practiced my favorite mantras, including "be still" and "I am."

Every time I felt like I had a handle on things, something would happen and I'd fall apart again. For the first time in years, I felt like I was a victim to everything happening around me and I was as stressed as I could remember being. What was most maddening though, was that deep down, I knew I didn't have to be feeling that way.

And, in case you had to ask, some of my old eating habits came roaring right back.

I was sitting outside on one of the first sunny days in March, writing in my journal. I felt as low as I had felt in years, and I was chronicling my complaints, my stresses and my frustrations. I kept asking myself "Why am I doing this to myself again?"

As I wrote, it occurred to me that there must be something I was getting from being stressed that was making me resist committing fully to changing. During my coaching training, we talked a lot about why someone might hesitate in the face of a change that they say they want. One quote from author Dr. Henry Cloud stuck with me: "We change our behavior when the pain of staying the same becomes greater than the pain of changing."

Even when we desperately want the end result, the change that it takes to get there is going to be difficult, and sometimes even painful. Our old ways of thinking are more familiar and comfortable, and they don't require any effort. One of my clients refers to her old ways of thinking as "the grooves in her brain." It is frustrating when you find yourself falling back into old habits, but it's important to remember that you've probably practiced the old ways of thinking for many, many years.

There can also be a surprising benefit to your stress. Being stressed, or worried, or upset can earn us attention from the people we love. Most people experience this as children: when you're upset, and you go running to your parents, what do they do? For many people, tears were met by hugs, sympathy and love. Maybe even food! (I recognize that this sadly isn't always the case for every child, but is often a typical childhood experience.)

Despite the fact that we *want* to let go of being stressed, being worried, being upset, that also means letting go of the sympathy, support and attention we get for being in this state. Not surprisingly, I think most people would rationally acknowledge that if they were more relaxed, happy and content that they would probably attract *more* people and more positive attention into their life. Clinging to old habits as a way to get attention is a subconscious behavior and reinforced by the instant gratification of attention and sympathy from others.

When I sat outside journaling in the midst of my storm cloud days, this thought struck me hard. It was a difficult confession to make to myself. I was upset, and I kept holding on to that emotion because, subconsciously, I wanted those I loved to recognize and validate my feelings. It felt good to have my friends confirm that my situation sucked, and to have my husband and my family acknowledge my pain. But then what?

Would that temporary sympathy or validation of my emotions be worth more than a long-lasting experience of being content and peaceful? I realized that I had to acknowledge what I was getting from being upset, and let go of it, if I ever wanted to make a permanent change. Understanding *why* you might be resisting change is as important as the process of change itself.

Surprisingly, there are plenty of reasons to resist change. Changing yourself can change your relationships with other people. You may feel pressure, real or imagined, from people in your life as you try to create change for yourself. You are not the only one who has become accustomed to your old patterns of thoughts and behaviors. Often people resist change without even realizing it because they are afraid of how their weight loss or behavior change might impact their friends and family. This is understandable, especially when you consider that food is often an important part of our social lives, our cultural ties and our family rituals.

If you feel like you are experiencing resistance from your friends or family, the best way to handle this is to address it as tactfully but directly as possible. Chances are, the people in your life who love you want you to be healthier and they may not even realize that they are making it harder for you, or they don't know the best way to support you. For instance, they may not know whether or not you want them to say something when they see you eating something that they assume is not healthy for you. Most people *want* to feel helpful and supportive. The best way to go about decreasing resistance from other people is to be open and honest about how they can support you and approach any opposition you perceive with curiosity.

For example, James was a client of mine whose spouse constantly scheduled things during the time that he had set aside to go the gym. He told me that he felt like she was sabotaging his weight loss efforts, but he didn't know how to address it. In a situation like this, it would be easy for him to have lost his patience and to have accused his spouse of the sabotage. It's very likely that if he had done this, she would have grown defensive and instead of having a conversation about it, there would have been a fight. I explained to him how approaching the issue with a sense of curiosity might allow him to explore where his wife was coming from, without triggering her defensiveness.

The next time the situation happened, he addressed it. He had plans to go to the gym after work, and his wife let him know she had made dinner plans with another couple and expected him to be there. He was ready.

He said to his wife, "Of course, I'll be there because I know it's important to you. But just out of curiosity, why did you schedule it for tonight when I had told you that I was going to the gym?" James reported to me that he had kept his tone very light, and spoke very calmly. His wife responded and said "Oh- well, I guess didn't realize that that was so important to you."

James replied to her, "It really is. I'm scared that my health is going to be affected by my weight, and that I'm going to have a heart attack one day and leave you and the kids. Going to the gym is the best way I can figure out to take care of myself, and ultimately you guys. I'd like to try and go three or four times a week."

His wife was silent on the other end for a minute before saying, "Of course. I'll try to pay better attention to your workout schedule from now on."

This didn't completely solve the issue, but it opened the door for more future conversations. It turned out his wife had been upset that James, who already worked a long day at the office, was spending even more time away from the family at the gym. Once she better understood his motivation, she eventually became his biggest cheerleader. James told me that he felt a little silly being so vulnerable, but ultimately he was thankful that he addressed his wife's resistance and gained her support in the long run.

Not only is support from your friends and family critical for creating long term change, but the accountability that comes from sharing your goals with other people will also help keep you on track. It can be intimidating to tell other people what you are doing, but ultimately having others know about your intentions will help you stay on track if you hit a setback.

Equally important as addressing resistance is acknowledging the support you are receiving from friends and family. Once you share your goals with others, pay attention to who backs you up and make sure to thank them. This is the best way to guarantee continued support! Support can come in all sorts of forms: it might be verbal encouragement, a gym partner, or someone who does the cooking and grocery shopping for you. It can even be something as simple as a friend who lets you choose the restaurant to go out to eat. Acknowledge when your friends or family are supporting you, and thank them for it. A little appreciation goes a long way in growing your cheering section.

Chapter 14: Inside Out Weight Management

I've been personally and professionally invested in the world of weight loss for over a decade and I've worked with hundreds of people. I have experienced, seen, heard or read about just about every weight loss strategy out there. I have seen and used some really effective strategies, I've seen some really dangerous ones and I've seen (and tried) ones that just make me laugh. For instance, there was the time my best friend talked me into the Cabbage Soup Diet. On day 2 we were to eat ONLY raw vegetables the entire day. We spent that day together on a 12 hour car ride from New York to North Carolina. Twelve hours with baggies full of carrots, broccoli, celery... every vegetable we could stand. Thankfully the sun was shining and our CD player was loaded up with great tunes, or else I am certain we would have strangled each other somewhere around the Mason-Dixon line!

I learned what the most effective way to lose weight is, but it took me years to figure out why using that strategy was so much easier for some people than others. Calorie reduction is the backbone of any effective weight loss plan. Understanding calories in and calories out is a surprisingly easy concept. There are numerous tools and resources to help you figure out how many calories are in the foods you're eating, and even more restaurants are making that information readily available.

Despite these tools and information being readily available, the majority of people who seek to implement this strategy still struggle, and many fail. Those who are successful often remain stuck in a holding pattern of trying to maintain control, "falling off the wagon", suffering the guilt, and then getting back on track, like I did. It's an exhausting process, and one I personally partook in for years before I figured out what the missing piece was.

For a very small percentage of my clients, once they know how many calories they need they are off and running. When I ask them if they're having any trouble meeting their calorie budgets, they look at me like I just asked them if the moon was made of cheese. Weight loss is simply a mathematical equation to them, and having someone show them the tools has unlocked the process for them.

They are the exception.

Most of my clients, despite fully grasping the concept of calorie reduction, still struggled with mastering it. They'd maintain control until night time and then the cravings would set in as they settled down to watch their favorite TV show. They'd do fine until they had a crisis happen at work or they had to attend a big potluck gathering. Like them, I joked about being a stress eater and laughed at the irony of eating 3 bowls of cereal while I watched *The Biggest Loser*. I compensated with exercise behaviors, or trying to be stricter, but it was constantly a struggle.

Understanding and implementing calorie reduction is often simply not enough to be successful at long-term weight maintenance. As I've mentioned many times throughout this book, all actions stem from our feelings. All our feelings stem from our thoughts. When we are struggling with our healthy choices, like exercising or making the best food decisions for ourselves, it is not willpower we lack. It is recognition that our thoughts are dictating those actions, by creating certain feelings. Constantly trying to change the actions, without any attention given to the thoughts that are behind them, will create that holding pattern of control, lapse, and guilt and back to control.

Albert Einstein once said the definition of insanity is doing the same thing over and over again and expecting different results. That Albert sure was one brilliant man. Trying to change your actions over and over again, without changing your thoughts, will get you the same results over and over again.

The key to changing your behavior is to change your thoughts.

Although it sounds very simple, it is extremely powerful. Changing your thoughts will in turn change how you are feeling. How you feel at any given moment will determine whether the choices that support a healthy weight come easily to you or feel like a struggle. For anyone who thinks they know what to do to lose weight, but find that they're constantly fighting themselves in the actual use of that knowledge, this is the missing piece.

The shift in my own thinking I described in the first chapter came as a surprise to me, but its effect has been long lasting and powerful. I had gotten to a point where I just assumed that I would always mentally struggle with how I felt about my body, food, and myself. I had been introduced to the idea of changing my thoughts to help grow my coaching business and I felt like I had nothing to lose by trying the same process out on how I felt about my weight. It was with a mixture of surprise and happiness that I wrote that journal entry over Christmas.

It has been almost five years since I wrote that journal entry where I committed myself to letting go of the fight. While I can't claim it has been a perfect journey without a single bump in the road, I have felt more content and peaceful over these last five years than I would have imagined possible. There have certainly been relapses and times where I felt overwhelmed by stress and unhappiness, but these have simply been opportunities to prove to myself again the power of changing my thoughts.

When I stopped fighting myself, I realized I had nearly effortlessly dropped 5 pounds and continued to remain stable at that weight. It was almost as if letting go of the mental weight allowed my body to release the physical weight. I no longer feel ruled by battles of emotional eating or the compelling need to balance out a bout of overeating with an equal amount of calorie burn through exercise. I've grown to appreciate and enjoy exercise for the act of doing it, instead of focusing on the number of minutes, miles or calories. That has been one of the biggest surprises! Most importantly, the constant chatter in my head that created feelings of guilt, inadequacy or self-recrimination about my food choices, my exercise, or my weight no longer plagues me.

I was also pleased to realize that the process of changing my thoughts and creating more positive, powerful experiences spilled over into other areas of my life. I felt more confident as I moved forward with my coaching business. I felt less fear and more abundance as I dealt with my finances, another area that I had always struggled with feelings of control and uncertainty. I still experience days or sometimes even month-long periods of stress or frustration in all of these areas, but even as I was in the midst of these periods the knowledge that I had the ability to get myself out of these bouts of despair by changing my thought process buoyed me and gave me confidence that anything I was going through would, at most, be a temporary experience.

This is what gets me most excited about sharing this process: knowing that once you apply it to your life for managing your weight, you will soon experience that you can apply it to *any* area of your life. I'm certain you picked up this book to learn how to master your weight management skills, but you have inadvertently picked up a guide to creating change in any area of your life. The process is exactly the same. Anywhere you want to change your behaviors, you must change your thoughts.

If you were to plant an orchard of apple trees, you would start with an apple seed. One day if you decided you'd prefer to see a change in your orchard, you wouldn't start with the fruit itself, or even the leaves, the branches or its thick, sturdy trunk. You would go right to the beginning: you would start with the seed. You must always remember that the seeds you plant determine what grows.

Once you recognize that your thoughts are the seeds that will change what fruit your life bears, you will understand that you have the power to create any kind of life experience that you want from the inside out.

Appendix

Questions to Identify Emotional Eating:

This is by no means an exhaustive list of questions nor is there a certain amount of "yes" or "no" answers that determine definitively whether or not you're eating for emotion reasons. These questions are not diagnostic, but are simply intended to explore your patterns of eating.

1. Did I consciously decide to eat this specific food or amount of food?

2. How do I feel while I'm eating? (Happy? Guilty? Disconnected? Relaxed? Stressed?)

3. How do I feel after I'm eating?

4. Is this certain food one I often reach for when I'm feeling stressed, overwhelmed, upset, etc.?

5. Is this a one-time event or repeat behavior?

6. Was I influenced by the choices of other people around me?

7. Is it a holiday? Is this food a family tradition or other social event?

8. Am I at an event that I usually associate with this type of food? (For example, popcorn at a movie theater or hot dogs at a sporting event.)

9. Was I drinking before I ate this food?

10. Am I overtired?

None of these questions alone can determine whether or not you were experiencing emotional eating, but they can help you to think about your food choices in greater detail. Sometimes what may seem like emotional eating is really a result of the influences of our social circle, traditions or habits. For instance, many people are in the habit of eating popcorn when they go to the movie theater and they may eat too much in one sitting and feel bad about it. However, despite the large portion sizes and the feelings of guilt, this might not be an example of emotional eating.

References

Perkinson, Richard. *Chemical Dependency Counseling: A Practical Guide.* Thousand Oaks: Sage Publications, 2011. Print.

Nelson-Jones, Richard. *Practical Counselling and Helping Skills.* London: Sage Publications, 2005. Print.

Thank You

My gratitude to those who helped this book come to fruition is boundless. I have been so fortunate to have so many people cheerlead, encourage and help me with this book.

Thank you to the great mentors and teachers I've had along the way who have helped me develop my writing or my understanding of behavior change. These include Sarah Nazarian, Lauren Updyke, Shannon Mihalko, Adam Levithan, Ed Decosta and Garry Lindsay.

Thank you to colleagues along the way who have traded ideas with me and helped me grow as a coach including Sam Rogers, Lauren Cook, Heather Dunn and Susan Johannesmann.

Thank you to those who edited the final editions of this including Sara Wilson and Tamara Scott.

Thank you to the many friends who encouraged me along the way with the project and told me they believed in me. There are too many of you to name, but just know every single time one of you complimented my writing or responded with enthusiasm to my ideas, you lifted me up.

Thank you to all the clients I've had along the way that have trusted me with their stories and allowed me to be part of their journeys.

Thank you to my Mom and Dad for their unconditional support in my writing, coaching skills and anything else

I've endeavored to try. Thank you to my siblings, Michael and Katie, for your interest and excitement and helping me flesh out ideas over many a glass of wine.

Thank you to my son Bowen for showing up in the world and giving me added inspiration. Thank you also for your extra long naps during those early months that allowed me to finish writing this.

Most importantly, thank you to my husband Matt. I can still remember sitting at lunch on vacation with you and mentioning that I wanted to write a book. Your response "So write a book!" was so confident, it was as if I had already done it. Thank you for your on-going support and interest in my project, but mostly your unwavering belief that I would be able to do it.

19723062R00063

Made in the USA
Lexington, KY
03 January 2013